7-Step Guide to
Speaking Success

AN ESSENTIAL HEALTHCARE LEADER'S HANDBOOK

By
Daniel Pennington

Foreword

By Quint Studer

Being a leader in healthcare today is harder than it has ever been. We're faced with constant change, shrinking margins, and enormous uncertainty. Our roles continue to evolve with a greater emphasis on improving patient outcomes through evidence-based care. At the heart of that care must be an effective communication strategy.

The complexity of the healthcare system means every step of patient care has to be coordinated with other people, other departments and often even other healthcare systems. Routinely a single patient's care can involve the logistics of planning and structuring care across multiple departments and institutions.

Into this complexity, we throw leaders who often have very little or no training. Those who survive are those who seek out additional resources and take their personal and professional development into their own hands. That's why I'm pleased you are reading this book. In every organization, we've seen it's easy to tell who the high performers are. They are the leaders who don't wait to be developed, they take responsibility for their careers and become lifelong learners. Reading and attending training will be crucial to our survival in the coming years.

The three most critical skills any healthcare leader needs are the ability to hire well, the courage to terminate an employee when necessary, and the determination to communicate at every level. I'm convinced you can never communicate too much, but the quality of that communication is vital.

Too often we are drowning in a sea of emails, meetings, and conference calls. We have too much information but too little communication. Separating noise from know-how is increasingly difficult. That's where "7-Step Guide to Speaking Success" becomes such a vital tool. What you are holding is a practical guide with a step-by-step process for your everyday communication.

Daniel has studied hundreds of healthcare leaders from across a broad swath of the industry, looking to discover those who are effective and why, and those who aren't and what they could stand to learn. Our time together at the Studer Group allowed him to spend time with some of the top healthcare executives at national conferences. Why does the audience cheer and applaud one leader and mostly ignore the next one? Why do viewers remember key takeaways from one presentation and find the next forgettable? Why does this leader come across as having charisma and authenticity? Why did this leader fail to capture the hearts of her employees even when it appears she is doing everything right?

This "7-Step Guide to Speaking Success" is full of tactical and practical information you can apply to your communications right away. From PowerPoint to compelling storytelling, from memorization to body language, the "7-Step Guide to Speaking Success" takes you on a deep dive into the mechanics and planning of a powerful presentation. I am confident you will find this guide an indispensable tool for preparing your next presentation.

-Quint Studer is the founder of The Studer Group and author of seven leadership-based books both inside and outside the healthcare industry. His books have landed on both the Wall Street Journal and Business Week's bestsellers list.

Preface

Communication mistakes are a twelve-billion-dollar headache for healthcare, which accounts for about half of the 3.8% profit margin. With that much money at stake, you would think communication training for healthcare leaders would be one of the first and most important areas of leadership development. Unfortunately, it is not.

How does a healthcare professional get to be a leader? In many instances, the boss is promoted or moves to another place of employment, and suddenly you find yourself in a supervisory role. Training for your new leadership responsibilities, if offered at all, might consist of a couple of books to read and learned experiences from your yearly evaluation conference. Overall, very few dollars are spent helping to make healthcare leaders better at communicating, even though communication is one of the most important skills a leader should possess.

Initiatives requiring useful communication skills often begin at the C-Suite level before being *communicated* to department's heads, which *communicate* with supervisors, who communicate with directors, who *communicate* with staff. At any point that these communications are of poor quality, your role as a leader is hampered, the initiative fails, employees become disengaged, and patient care can suffer.

Healthcare leaders spend eighty percent of their day communicating. So how are they doing?

Studies from McKinsey Global Institute, International Data Corporation, and the Journal of Communication suggest a healthcare leader spends up to eighty percent of their day communicating. Small to medium-sized businesses spend about seventeen hours a week *clarifying* weak and ineffective communication at an average cost per business of more than a half-million dollars annually.

The problem goes well beyond the walls of healthcare. A 2014 study by About.com determined that poor communication accounted for the top three reasons people do not like their jobs. Respondents mentioned lack of clear direction, lack of clarity relative to their job performance, and constant change that isn't well communicated.

Unclear expectations. Poor communication causes employees to question their job responsibility and position within the company. They do not know what is expected of them or what they need to do to succeed. They fill their days with second-guessing and distrust of their managers. Sound familiar?

Rumor and gossip. Employees seek to fill the communications void with rumor and gossip. They look for 'signs' of what might be happening and work to fill in the blanks. Executives perceived as 'looking worried' might mean layoffs are coming. Strangers in suits might mean a merger is imminent. In fact, analyses of work environments indicate that gossip is a prominent sign of ineffective or nonexistent communication in an organization.

Performance issues. Without clear communication job performance suffers. Deadlines are missed, and roles are confused. Employees may take too long on trivial tasks and delay starting or even avoid other, more crucial activities. Being productive requires clear communication of goals for the organization and expectations for the individual. If employees are forced to guess what is expected of them because these things are not adequately communicated to them, they often will get it wrong.

Customer service effects. As bad as under-communication is for the organization, it is customer service, which suffers the most. Missed promises to the employee and the customer lead to resentment toward the chain of command from both groups. Customer service is a team activity, requiring everybody to be on board. Without clear communication, a complaint can get pushed from department to department, which further exacerbates negative feelings. A team that communicates clearly to the team members and the public, which it serves, reduces the number of issues in the first place and resolves problems faster.

Turnover results. The net effect of poor communication within the organization is employee turnover. After all, who wants to work for a group that has unclear goals and roles, that encounters directives for change without clear expectations, that struggles with gossip and rumor, and that continually deals with poor customer service issues? An employee in this perpetually shifting environment, with no clear direction for improvement, begins to look elsewhere for work.

It's not surprising then that "communication skills" are the number one most-wanted set of abilities for new hires. What can be done, though, for leaders who are already in the system?

The Good News
The good news is that the ability to communicate effectively and proficiently is a learned set of skills. In our classes around the country, we see healthcare leaders dramatically improve their communication in a short period, once they learn to focus on the necessary skills. This book has been written to help guide you through that process.

Healthcare requires individuals to engage in complex interactions, through both the spoken and written word and using both personal and technological applications. In almost every instance, no matter how minor, the activities must be coordinated within a handful if not a hospital full of people. Successful leaders will tell you that the only way to always align these activities is through constant, consistent and highly effective communication.

Many people think of communication skills as applied only to such unique experiences as public speaking. For them, having to speak to a group means preparing and presenting a speech to a vast assemblage of strangers. It may imply a lectern, microphone, large room, maybe a video camera, and lots of people. Also, for many of those people, the scene conjures up a healthy dose of stage fright.

No wonder most leaders within an organization say they never engage in public speaking. The reality is that most do not, like that at least. However, they do provide information to their co-workers during department meetings. They do engage with the public when extending the mission of the organization. They do communicate with those who supervise them or those whom they manage as part of the organization's daily give-and-take. They literally 'speak' for a living, but because there is not a stage and a microphone it somehow does not count. All of these leader roles require the same level of effective communication skills as the public speaker, just in a different context.

> *Speaking is speaking whether to a handful of coworkers in a huddle or to strangers in a conference ballroom. The same skills are still needed, and the same consequences are at stake.*

Within this book we'll discuss strategies for engaging your audience, clarifying your message, speaking from the heart, being authentic, using stories and other methods to make your content memorable and effective. Once learned, these skills will be useful in small groups, around a conference room table, during one-on-one sessions, and even within emails.

> *Clear, compelling communication is key to your success and the success of your organization. You owe it to your staff, your organization, and most importantly to your patients and their families to provide superior communication at every level every single day.*

Daniel Pennington, 2018

Table of Contents

Preface 7
Step One 17
Diagnose Before You Treat 17
Step Two 33
   Start Strong 33
Step Three 49
   The WHY Formula 49
Step Four 71
   Storytelling Basics 71
Step Five 87
   Rules of Engagement 87
Step Six 163
   Show Some Statistics 163
Step Seven 169
   Finish Strong 169
Bonus Chapter 179
   PowerPoint Success 179
   Bonus Chapter 213
   All of This is Worthless 223
   Final Thoughts 229
Acknowledgments 239

Step One
Diagnose Before You Treat

Before we begin working on any presentation we need to understand:

- Our subject
- Our goals
- Our audience
- Our manager's expectations

When we begin constructing our presentation without first answering some of these fundamental questions our chances for success are pretty low.

> *If you don't know where you are going, any road will get you there. -Lewis Carol*

What is your manager expecting from this presentation?

When I was a young manager, my immediate supervisor insisted I communicate lengthy initiative to my staff. The problem was my staff only met once a month, and our meetings had to be kept to under a half hour. I remember running through the content at lightning speed. I'm guessing my staff felt overwhelmed by the material, but truthfully, I never noticed their faces, I was too intent on covering everything. I looked up; confident I had done my duty and dismissed my staff with a precious few minutes to spare. Do you think anyone indeed learned anything? Of course not.

The fire hose does not work. We've seen far too many leaders begin with dozens of slides, hundreds of bullet points, and enough content to fill an encyclopedia. They then try to cram all of that into a thirty-minute presentation. They sometimes proclaim confidently, "I can *cover* all of this." The question isn't how much *you can cover;* the problem is how much can your audience *receive and retain*? *Listening* is hard work. *Remembering* and being able to *act on* the information is even harder.

Effective communication does not involve drowning your audience in a Niagara Falls of facts. The audience needs to hear and understand what you are saying, put that into their own words, figure out how that connects to information they already know, and then decide where to store this new information.

If your points are meant to replace information they already know, they have the additional work to judge your new information, decide that it supersedes what they already know, remove the existing information and replace it with the original. That involves many steps, and we shouldn't shortchange the amount of mental energy that it takes. Now imagine this entire process is repeated a few dozen times in an hour. Listening is, indeed, hard work.

So, we begin by managing expectations. In a given time frame we can only effectively communicate a given amount of information. When supervisors or managers have unrealistic expectations, they frustrate leaders and confuse employees.

What type of presentation will it be? We communicate most effectively when our communication goals align with our presentation type. A two-day long workshop naturally can effectively communicate more information than a twenty-minute huddle.

A huddle is a brief, informal, often standing presentation meant to communicate immediate information to a small team.

A talk is an informal communication that rarely lasts more than a half hour. The expectation is to create a casual atmosphere and communicate a few simple ideas in a friendly approachable format.

A presentation is a more formal affair, usually attended by a larger group and held in a more formal space. Quite often a presentation involves some form of PowerPoint or slides, introductions, and handouts. Presentations are longer than a talk, usually lasting for more than an hour with scheduled breaks. Presentations can often cover quite a bit of material and, when coupled with handouts and follow-up written communications, can be useful for communicating complex information.

A workshop is usually defined by the amount of audience involvement that is expected. Workshops can be short, as brief as an hour, or can stretch over several days. Workshops are excellent for communicating information that later will need to be acted upon. The presenter or trainer will spend some time training and then follow up with a practice session that the audience participates in. The process takes considerably more time than a presentation, but the audience learns more deeply than if they are merely casual observers.

The keynote. Keynotes are often the most formal of all presentations. They can be grand affairs with thousands of people in the audience and are usually held in magnificent ballrooms outfitted with chandeliers and soft music. Most commonly the keynote's purpose is to inspire and elevate the audience. These speakers can be paid presenters earning thousands of dollars, or the very highest echelon of CEOs from the loftiest C-Suite in the organization. Many times, the actual information communicated will take a back seat to inspiring messages meant to win the hearts and minds of the audience.

It's a good idea, to begin with, the consideration of the type of presentation you will be giving. That is often dependent on your end goal. Do you need to inspire an entire organization to embrace change and set sail for a new future? That's a keynote. If you are training and you have sufficient time, you would be well-served to choose a workshop.

Regardless of the type of presentation, you are planning; you will be more successful if you try to communicate less information. The firehose does not work. Cut your information in half and then cut it again.

Each point will need sufficient time to explain. Perhaps you will need examples. You may want the audience to practice this new information. They may have questions about each point. You may need to tell a story to illustrate each point. Then it would be wise to check in with them to make sure they've gotten each point. "Did you get that? Now does that make sense?" "What questions come to your mind as you process these ideas? What do we need to clarify?" "Are there some dots we have not connected yet for you? Which ones?"

So, the formula includes:

- New idea
- Examples
- A story about the new idea
- Audience practice
- Questions and answers

- *Check in to validate learning*

This formula might take ten to twelve minutes per idea, so in a half-hour presentation, you might only have time for two or three ideas. Remember: the goal is for the audience to hear/learn/retain/be able to act on the idea, not how quickly you can speak. Covering a topic is not the same as teaching that topic. Our effectiveness gauge must measure how much the audience *learns,* not just how much they've been *exposed* to the ideas.

Pairing different types of communication can enhance your effectiveness. If your talk is technical, you may want to send the audience home with a handout or practice exercises. After all, remembering the complex information later can be augmented by printed material in the form of diagrams, summaries, and outlines. If you want to inspire and elevate, you may be able to supplement your talk with posters placed in the breakroom. Regardless, a follow-up email with crucial takeaways usually reinforces your message. Sometimes audience members will ask for a copy of your slides. However, if you create your slide deck well, your slides may not be all that useful later. See Chapter 14 for more PowerPoint training.

The jug-and-mug does not work either

I'll slip in another metaphor here, the jug-and-mug. At some point, people have imagined the teacher as a jug full of knowledge and the students as empty mugs waiting to be filled. The jug-teacher wanders through the room pouring out her expertise into the receptive mug-students.

I cannot speak for elementary students, but I know adult learners are not empty vessels waiting to benefit from our genius. In fact, the very idea seems inconsiderate. Our "students" are fully-functioning intelligent adults who already know a great deal and may be smarter than we are. As we try to teach them, we must realize they likely already have a basic understanding of your topic, or they wouldn't be there in the first place. They will only learn from you if they deem the new information as *worthy of their time* and *valuable to their lives*. They 'judge' the content from the jug-teacher and are not ready to open their mug-minds until we demonstrate the value of what we are saying.

- Audience member one asks: "What's in this for me?"
- Audience member two asks: "Please don't overwhelm me!"

- Audience member three asks: "How can you solve my problem right now?"

Have one good idea

Every good presentation is an outgrowth of one good idea. A presentation is a structured, planned event, meant to convey a carefully thought through an idea with clarity. A clear idea begets a clear presentation, and a vague idea begets a vague presentation. That said, this is not the time to ruminate about the exact parameters of your idea. You can be loose here and tighten up later. Let's get something down on paper and see what we can do with it. In a hospital context some ideas might be:

1. Reducing patient anxiety requires constant clear communication at all levels.
2. Aligned teams outperform misaligned teams.
3. Excellent patient care begins before the patient ever arrives at our door.

Your idea may be relatively specific and unique but take a minute and write it down. It does not have to be beautiful at this point because you'll have time to polish it later.

Start incredibly broad

The best initial research is wide-ranging and playful.

If your topic is about how humans learn, you may want to research how primates learn or how the ancient Chinese learned. You may be interested in great learning failures or the oldest colleges in the world. You may find it interesting to research learning disabilities or how people with specific brain problems struggle to learn. Don't do your research and dig only in one area. The sweet spot for your final presentation may be miles away from where you begin.

Sticky notes are your friend

A helpful technique in building your presentation is the use of a blank wall and sticky notes. Jot each note, chart, factoid, and quote on a separate note. They do not have to be complete; it can be as simple as "Limits of rounding, what we do not know." Then place the notes into a rough order on the wall. Move them around into another order. Do you see your big idea yet? Soak up all the information. Argue with your content and try to make it fit your preconceived notions. Peruse each note over and over. Does this belong to that one? Are these two notes redundant? Is this one out of place no matter where you put it? It will become clear what idea should be grouped, which ideas need more support, and which ideas you do not need at all. Play with various structures. Regroup things that feel better together. Use this time to remove things that do not fit.

Look outside the box

The best ideas are likely to come from traditional outside sources. If you are researching the subject of *learning*, and you only consider *how we learn in schools*, you are unlikely to develop an idea that is new and refreshing. If, however, you step back and realize we are always learning all of the time and we are only occasionally learning in a school environment you'll miss a plethora of other concepts. Why, for instance, is a child who is considered by his teachers to have attention deficit disorder able to master an elaborate video game like Titanfall or Falcon 3? If you are researching professional development, you may find that professional athletes who are at the top of their league still receive hours of coaching every week. If you study a Renaissance artist like Rembrandt, you find he often had dozens of skilled artists as students.

I have a box of random ideas - now what?

Don't write your presentation yet. Random ideas cannot be melded into a winning presentation any easier than grabbing the next seven people you meet and blending them into a boy band.

What does your audience already know about this subject?

I've been lucky to work with the team at Studer Community Institute and every time I step onto the stage I already know a great deal about the people I will be speaking to. How? SCI always creates a *pre-conference survey*. These dozens or so questions give us tremendous feedback on how much the audience already knows about the subject. We also ask what their biggest challenge is, what they hope to learn, and any questions they need to be answered. By carefully crafting my message to exactly their stated needs and concerns we have a much higher chance of success.

The other question, which is vital to understand, is *how receptive this audience* to this information is? Most people in healthcare are 'full-plate' people. They are overwhelmed with duties already, and when our presentation seems to contain just one more assignment to stack on top of their task list, they understandably resist. Change is hard for anyone. Change can feel impossible for people who are already overwhelmed. Unless we present our information as helping to take some tasks off their plates, we may find the audience unreceptive or even hostile to our ideas.

I remember a conversation with a nurse leader from Australia. She was almost shell-shocked from a presentation that didn't go well. When we looked through her slide deck, it was something like, "Twelve things you **must do** when rounding on a patient." I remember her telling me, "They booed me! I've never been booed before!" Luckily, we were able to revise her presentation to focus on how much time hourly rounding saves rather than listing what appeared to be a dozen new tasks. Her new slide deck which emphasized time-saving was much better received.

What are your goals for this presentation?

What do you want your audience to think, do or feel as a result of seeing your presentation? Answering this question before you begin working on your presentation is critical. Different presentations have different goals.

The inspirational message

We all love the inspirational message, and honestly, I don't think anyone experiences enough of them. Dr. Martin Luther King, Jr., Anthony Robbins, Les Brown, Zig Ziglar are heroes in my book. So much of the life of healthcare professionals can be challenging that when confronted with an inspirational message we all brighten a bit. In business, however, inspiration often takes a back seat to information.

The informational message

The majority of all talks we give are merely informational. Think of a shift-change huddle or a progress report presented at a department head meeting. The utilitarian nature of the informational speech, however, doesn't preclude our responsibility to make it enjoyable. The purpose of the informative speech is to inform, impart knowledge, clarify, and create understanding.

The persuasive message

The purpose of the persuasive speech is to get the audience to do something. We often have to overcome objections, prove our contentions are well-founded and make sound arguments for our suggestions.

The reality is most of the time we deliver a message that contains components of all of these types. Look in Chapter 3 to see how the "Why" formula manages to make your message persuasive, informative, and inspirational all at once.

Step Two
Start Strong

Your first seven seconds

In your first seven seconds of speaking, your audience will decide whether to sit forward and listen or sit back and forget you. Research from *Rate My Professor* reveals this seven-second rule. The researchers took seven-second video clips of top-rated teaching professors and seven-second videos of worst-rated teaching professors. Mixing up the order of videos, the researchers asked a panel to view the video clip of each professor with the sound off. The group was then asked to guess which professors were the best and which the worst. Each time, the panel correctly guessed those who were top-rated and those who scored at the bottom.

In seven seconds an audience figures out whom they like and whom they do not like. They quickly decide who is worth watching, who is worth ignoring, who not to miss and whom to avoid. So, what should you do in your first seven seconds? Unfortunately, most speakers fill up their first seven seconds with unnecessary words like these:

> "Thank you, John, for inviting me. Thank you, Martha, for that warm introduction. When your Vice Chairman suggested I speak to you today, we talked about your company and some of your challenges. That's why I'm delighted to have this chance to be here even if the weather isn't cooperating. What about that game last night? Huh. Wasn't that a great game?"

You are now two or three minutes into your presentation and still, have not said anything of substance. Begin close to the action

The Star Trek Open

Remember Star Trek? Their starship would fly across galaxies, soar through universes, zoom past planets and finally beam down. Where would they beam down? One rock away from where the action is. Your opening statement should do the same. Begin as close as possible to the action of your story. No build up. No filler phrases or wasted setups. Bam! Your first line should start right in the middle of the good stuff. Here are a few opening lines from some very successful TED Talks:

"As we climbed to three thousand feet the plane suddenly shuddered. I heard a loud pop and smoke appeared in the galley."

"I do not want to alarm anyone, but the person to your left is a liar."

"Sadly, in the next eighteen minutes, while I speak, four Americans who are alive now will be dead because of the food they will eat today.

"Today, you will learn something that will add ten years to your life."
"Twenty years from now, your job won't exist."

"Did you know more people have access to a mobile phone than a toilet?"

The Question Open

An intriguing open engages the audience and gets them to sit forward and listen rather than leaning back and playing Angry Birds. A surprising way to snag attention is to ask a provocative question.

- What if you were George Bailey in "It's a Wonderful Life," and you could experience what your world would look like without you in it. What do you think would be the most significant change?
- Researchers studied groups who lived past 100 years old and found a startling paradox. What personality trait do you think is most strongly correlated with living that long?
- If left-handedness is strongly associated with mental illness, alcoholism, and early death, why hasn't left-handedness died out?

The early question sets up the audience to listen for the answer. We all love puzzles and mental challenges so by starting your talk with the central mystery your speech will unravel we find ourselves engaged in the journey. Puzzles work even better if you can 'try out' and dismiss a few possible solutions along the way.

- Why does left-handedness persist?
- These researchers suggest a genetic link. However, then how do you explain identical twins that are different-handed?
- Maybe it's birth-trauma. However, there is no substantial connection between

difficult birth and the eventual handedness of the child.

As you set up and then debunk various explanations, the listeners dive deeper and deeper into the mystery until you finally release the tension by revealing the answer.

The Quotation Open

> "Walter Cronkite said 'the current healthcare system is neither healthy, caring or a system.'"

We use quotes to gather the shared credibility of the person you choose to quote. The audience might quibble with *your* analysis of the healthcare system, but they would struggle to impugn the credibility of the beloved CBS news anchor Walter Cronkite. Beginning your presentation with a quote can be powerful but only if the quote fully encapsulates the message in your talk and that is sometimes a tall order.

A quote that *sort of* works, but *not precisely*, might send your audience's attention in a different direction and you might spend much time trying to bring them back. The above quote by Walter Cronkite might work correctly for a presentation about challenges in our current system but might distract from a discussion of financial regulations concerning Accountable Care Organizations. Choose carefully.

The Startling Statistic Open

> "The United States spends 3.2 billion dollars a year on healthcare or roughly ten-thousand dollars per person. To put that into perspective, that is thirty percent more than any other developed country, and more than twice as much as Germany, Canada, Australia, France, Japan or the United Kingdom."

Our audience is asking, "Why should I care about this presentation?" Answering with a startling statistic from the beginning does a great job of explaining that. That massive number is so large it overwhelmingly explains the value of this presentation.

There is one caution, however. The first few seconds of a presentation are often a 'settling in' period for the audience. People may still be putting their purses away, getting out a pen and paper and starting to focus their attention. It is often good to set up your startling statistic with a brief sentence or two:

> "Healthcare is expensive, right? Also, that's true of no matter where in the world you need it. Healthcare is expensive in every country, isn't it? Well actually...the United States spends 3.2 billion dollars a year on healthcare or roughly ten-thousand dollars per person."

The set up bridges a person's attention as they settle in to listen.

The Story Open

> "At the other end of the hallway, my father lay dying. His eighty-two-year-old heart betrayed him. His cells struggled for oxygen. His kidneys were shutting down. A solemn nurse spoke in a soft voice to my brother and me. You should go, she said, and say your goodbyes. I still had my car keys in my hand, and some part of me wanted to just leave, to just drive away. And that day no one would have blamed me."

A compelling story immediately grabs your audience and tells them that something new is happening. It says this is not your usual talk. The audience responds by giving you their complete attention.

We cannot overemphasize the importance of your open. People will remember your open and your close. If you make the open and close powerful enough the other sections of your talk can be more forgettable, and you will still be effective. In our one-on-one training, we spend a vast majority of our time and energy on the open because we understand capturing the attention of an audience is key to your presentation's success.

Be adventurous with your story structure

You will be tempted to present information chronologically. Saying how this happened first, then this, and finally that. While there is nothing wrong with a strict chronological order, it does not have the impact of a more ambitious structure. A more effective opening, employing a cinematic structure, begins right in the middle of the biggest challenge. Here is the first sentence from a well-known hospital CEO:

> *"Six weeks into my tenure at the hospital I realized we were bankrupt."*

This CEO went on to explain various attempts to restructure finances, and every time a new plan was thought to save them, that plan failed. This speaker's audience sat on the edge of their seats wondering how the hospital would eventually survive.

Chronological Structure
- The first thing we did
- The second thing we did
- The third thing we did
- Results
- Success

Cinematic Structure
- Impending disaster
- Failed attempts to solve the problem
- Employees jump ship
- Crazy idea
- Success

A cinematic structure creates and releases tension several times over the course of a presentation. We are accustomed to this structure in movies (hence the name, cinematic) where a hero finds trouble and gets out of it, only to find problem again. Think of a James Bond film where Bond is nearly killed in the first few minutes of the film but escapes, only to see himself in trouble again. As the conflict with the antagonist intensifies, our hero encounters increasing difficulties, fleeing again and again. This constant tension compels the audience to lean forward and not take their eyes off the screen.

Create a burning platform

A great many times the purpose of speaking is to affect change. Our team, for instance, is currently doing things one-way and we need to convince them to do things a different way. However, change is hard for everyone. How then do we approach an audience who resists change? Quite often we use the burning platform.

> *At 9:30 p.m. on a July evening in 1988, the crew of the Piper Alpha oil-drilling platform in the North Sea off the coast of Scotland heard an explosion. Fire swept across the platform and engulfed the entire rig. Another more massive explosion blew through the firewalls and shot flames the length of the oilrig, killing one hundred and sixty-two crewmembers and two rescuers.*
>
> *Andy Mochan, a supervisor, stood at the edge of the platform and was faced with a terrible choice. He could choose certain death from the fire, or he could jump into the blackness of the North Sea and likely be pulled under to his death. "It was either fry or jump," he concluded, deciding the cost of staying would be too high, so he chose to*

dive into the unknown. Andy and a handful of others were the only ones to survive the disaster.

For many of us as trainers, the burning platform provides the best analogy for people to understand the cost of resisting change. Front load this burning platform analogy early in your presentation so that your audience will understand what's in it for them.

Creating and then releasing tension is engaging. Unfortunately, if we aren't careful, we can rob our stories of tension. I'll give you an example: Debbie, a nurse leader, told the above story about Andy and the burning platform. However, she *began* her story with, "Andy jumped into the North Sea, preferring as he said, to possibly die from drowning rather than certainly die from the fire." She then went on to describe the explosion, the fire, and how Andy ended up on the edge of the platform. Told like this, backward, with the conclusion first, the story lacked any tension and therefore wasn't engaging. Don't rob your story of its tension! Focus on the moment of choice does he jump or not...and keep your audience on pins and needles as long as possible.

Use the words We and Your

No matter who your audience is they are only interested in themselves. As early as possible tell the audience how this topic affects *them*. Use the words we, *you, your,* and *our* frequently. Include them in your descriptions and examples, emphasizing how these instances will change *them*. Tell them the results *they* will feel or how we will feel. Tell them what *they* can do. Tell them how concerned *they* should be. Say it's *you*, and *yours*.

Connect with your audience with "we" and "our."

Sometimes the word 'you' can sound too bossy, too preachy. At those times a better choice can be 'we.' Listen to the way this changes the sentence:

> When rounding on <u>your unit you should</u>...
> When rounding on <u>our unit we should</u>...

There is a magic to the words we, our and us. At a recent training session in Nashville, I heard the nurse leader say:

> "As **you** go into the patient's room **you** should do **your** environmental assessment. **You'll** need to check bed rails to see if they

> *are up, and **you'll** need to make sure the patient can easily reach the call light."*

By merely changing "you" to "we" you are communicating the same information without the preachy overtones. Notice:

> *"As **we** go into the patient's room **we'll** do **our** environmental assessment. **We'll** need to check bed rails to see if they are up, and **we'll** need to make sure the patient can easily reach the call light."*

Do you remember how I began this book?

> "In the next five years, eighty-five percent of your success will have to do with your ability to speak and communicate your ideas. Eighty-five percent. That's more than your degree. That's more than the years we've spent in the industry. That's more than your connections. Eighty-five percent of our success in the next five years is dependent on our ability to speak and communicate our ideas."

Nine times in that short piece I used the words we, your, or our.

Take a stand

No one wants to attend a weak, overly cautious presentation. Half-hearted speeches do not serve anyone, especially your audience. What if they disagree with your premise? Even better! An audience who challenges you is an audience that is engaged. Adult learners do not want to be spoon-fed information. They want, and demand, to be a part of the process. Pushback is essential to learning.

Children are accustomed to writing down whatever their teacher says and repeating it back on tests as if it were the absolute truth. Columbus "discovered" America, but not really. This continent was populated by millions of people for thousands of years before Columbus. Citing him as the discoverer of America may fit the rhyme and the tradition, but students remember this as if fact. Adults understand this is one person's take on the subject and while it might be correct, it might also be faulty. They reserve the right to disagree.

Imagine you are attending a conference that offers these two presentations at the same time. Which one most peaks your interest?

Your job will not exist in twenty years - how to survive when robots take over patient care.

Implications of artificial intelligence in healthcare.

Take a stand with your big idea. Be bold, but remember, your *big idea* is only *one thing*, not a dozen things. Get rid of extraneous ideas and hone your idea down to its bare essence. Chris Anderson, President of TED Talks, says,

> *"Even though these speakers and their topics all seem completely different, they actually do have one key common ingredient and it's this: Your number one task as a speaker is to transfer into your listeners' minds an extraordinary gift; a strange and beautiful object that we call an idea."*

Step Three
The WHY Formula

Finding your Why

During this training, I know you want results, and you want them fast. I hear, "Daniel, I'm busy. Why don't you tell me what to say and I'll say it."? That's where the *why formula* comes in.

I wouldn't call it magic, but it certainly has much power. While every presentation is unique, in my experience this formula works particularly well in the majority of cases. It goes something like this:

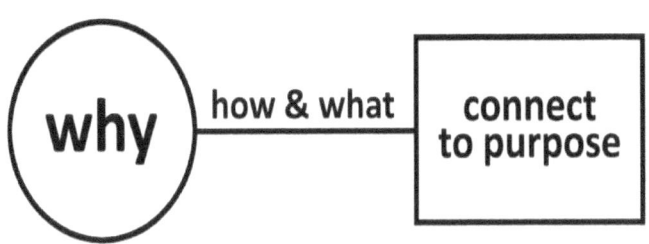

You start with your *why*, move on to your *how* and *what*, then finish with a *connect to purpose* story.

When I talk about the *why* what I mean is this: *Why do you do what you do? Why does your organization exist?* Sure, your company exists to make a profit, but does it also exist for a higher purpose than only making money? Do you, an employee, have a mission that goes beyond just collecting a paycheck at the end of the week? That is your *why*.

Years ago, researchers hired a study group to move bricks. Well paid, the group members were instructed to move heavy bricks from one side of a parking lot to the other. Then they were told to move the bricks back to the original side. If a member asked, they were told there was no purpose, no meaning, and no need for them to do the work. *Even though they were well paid,* most members quit within two days. The longest anyone worked was two weeks. As humans, we have a tremendous need to have a purpose. That sense of purpose, the knowledge that what we do matters, is your *why*.

This can be difficult to get your mind around. For instance, if you're an EMT and you save lives on a regular basis, you know what your *why* is. If you work in a hospital and you make life-and-death decisions for your patients, you understand what your *why* is. If you are a teacher anywhere in the education field, you also know precisely what your *why* is.

In many cases, your *why* is the reason you join or start a business in the first place. You may not always remember or think about it at the end of the day, but you understand there is a reason *why* you are in your line of work.

This is the good news about being in the healthcare field. Your *why* is front and center every day. Every time the bell rings on the pediatric unit and a child reaches another recovery milestone in their bout with cancer; you remember your why. Every time a car wreck victim is alert and talking when greeting his or her family, you understand your *why*. Every time a patient is discharged to return home to the regular routines of life, you know your *why*.

> *In our communications, we need to remind people of their why every time. A mission drives committed behavior; a task drives simple compliance.*

Regardless of your position within your organization, you work in service to a larger, greater good. Whether your role is behind the scenes handling payroll or out-front engaging with customers, the *organization's mission* is *your mission*.

During World War II when American soldiers drove tanks and flew planes into the German blitzkrieg, there were millions of Americans back home working hard to make the war effort succeed. For every soldier and sailor in harm's way, people were supporting them, in procurement, human resources, finance, in all sorts of jobs critical to Allied success. Victory could not have been achieved without the dedicated work and sacrifices of those who stayed behind.

If you're on the team, you get the win.

In the Vietnam War, there were twenty people in a support role for every one person with a rifle. If you were one of those support people, the military mission was your mission. Just because a soldier did not drive a tank, it did not mean he or she was not part of the mission.

It bears repeating:

If you're on the team, you get the win.

Also, this bears repeating, too. Regardless of your role in the effort, from the design team that plans the facility, to the bricklayers who labor to build, to the steelworkers who manufacture the construction materials, to the janitors who mop and wax the floors, to the universities and technical schools who train the staff, to the supervisors and secretaries who engage in the daily functions, all ultimately have a share in the team effort. Human endeavors are complex, and every worthwhile pursuit depends on dozens if not hundreds of other people to make it happen.

If you're on the team, you get the win.

The *Why formula* can be used in the context of a simple, brief conversation at Chuck E Cheese, in a break room discussion, or it can be expanded to work as a keynote. It's also useful for team meetings and hiring conversations. Once everyone understands the company is mission-driven, he or she will have a better buy-in to that mission.

In class, I often hear someone say, "But I'm just a _____." I interpret this to mean that they do not believe their role in the organization is significant enough to warrant this kind of communication training. Perhaps, though, they mean that their *work* is not important to the *mission* of the organization. Could it be that they are not yet convinced that they are part of a team doing mission-driven work? That this work takes everybody to make it happen? In a mission-driven, team-based organization, there is no such thing as "just a ___." We are all essential, for if any part fails, we run the risk of the mission failing. When the mission succeeds, everyone shares in the success, because each worker has contributed skills necessary to the effort. The work we do is vital, or we would not have been hired.

Author Simon Sinek talks a lot about the *why*. He has many books and videos you can view online about finding your *why* and starting with your *why*. Sinek teaches the *why* as the interior core of how we make decisions. As remarkable as Simon Sinek is at explaining the *why* connection, it appears to miss one particular thing. What do you do if your job does not have a *why*? Not every job is mission-driven. Not every job is even a *good* job. So, what happens then? Where do you find your *why* at that point? Let me introduce you to someone I know, Mr. Green.

Meet Mr. Green

On a recent trip to the campus of Florida Gulf Coast University, I called ahead to ask about parking and was instructed to stop at the entry gate and speak with the parking attendant, Mr. Green. At 7:00 a.m. the next morning I arrived at the nondescript guard shack. A tall, strapping, military-like man stepped out of the hut with the biggest smile I've ever seen. He reached out his hand, which was as big as a football player's, to shake mine and said, "Today is going to be a great day. How do I know it's going to be a great day? Because we're going to decide right now that you are going to have a great day." I replied, "Thank you, Mr. Green, can I please get a parking pass?" He did not let go of my hand. He continued, "No, you've got to say it - *today is going to be a great day.*" So, I repeated back to him, "Today is going to be a great day." Still, he held my hand, "Sir, you have to say it like you mean it - *today is going to be a great* day." Finally, I recited it back to him with his same enthusiasm, and he let me go, and I got my parking pass. I had never experienced *that* before.

Once on campus, I had a morning full of meetings, including an interview with the university president, and was asked to join several members for lunch. During our lunchtime conversation, I asked what was with this Mr. Green. Mr. Green retired from the Marines, but not ready to slow down, and he came to work at the University as their parking attendant.

"Mr. Green isn't *just* the parking attendant," the University President said. "He's more like the heartbeat of this university. People drive on campus every day to speak to Mr. Green. Students take their parents to meet him. People honk when they drive by and Mr. Green waves and smiles back. He is *the face* of FGCU because he is the first person most people meet when they visit our school."

I then learned about a time when the university realized Mr. Green had not taken any time off, so they forced him to take a vacation. When others noticed his absence, some speculated he had retired, and others thought he might be sick. Some even wondered if Mr. Green had died. "I had people in my office crying about Mr. Green," the University President said. "I had to write a memo to the staff explaining that Mr. Green was just on vacation."

Why do I tell you this story? Because many times in our work, we know precisely what our *why* is. If you're a doctor, nurse or educator, you have no trouble talking about your *why*. Sometimes, however, like Mr. Green, your *why* isn't what the job brings to you. Your *why* is what *you* bring to the task.

Mr. Green

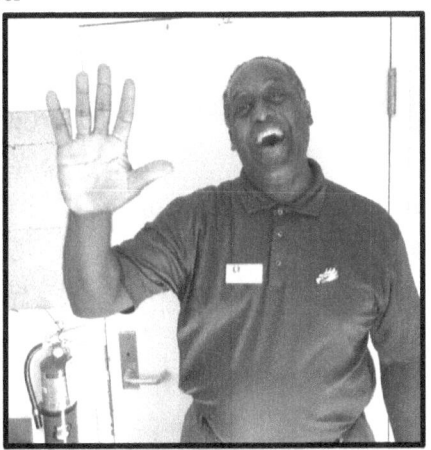

Move on to your How and What

Once you've clearly articulated your why, *it's time to move on to your* how *and* what. *Knowing your* how *and* what *is usually not too complicated since this is typically your focus every day. My caution to you, however, is this:*

> *People are not that interested in your how and what.*

Most people are interested in themselves, and they are only interested in your presentation since it can help them. That said your *how* and *what, that is, the workings of your organization,* do not directly impact their lives.

If you are inside an organization, you know a great deal about the how and what of that organization. How it is structured. How it finds customers. What the billing model is. What credentials the organization has. How many employees it has. On and on and on. How much of this does your audience need to know? The reality is very little. *You* find it interesting. *Your manager* finds it interesting. However, your audience glazes over very quickly, guaranteed.

If you don't believe me try this experiment: find a person who does not work for the same company as you. Tell them you are going to explain how your company works and what exactly it does. Ask them to raise their hand *the second* they get bored. Chances are your 'audience' won't get past a few minutes of hearing the details of the inner workings of your organization before they raise their hands. It just not that interesting to anyone who isn't directly involved in the organization.

That said you'll need to keep the details very short to sustain their attention. For example,

Your *why* might be:

> At Blue Hills Free Clinic, we believe everyone should have access to dental services, not just those who can afford to pay.

You then move to your *how* and *what,* which inevitably will have complexities, which you think, are essential, but this is not the time to elaborate on those details. Make it brief and move on.

> That's why we created a free dental clinic to serve disabled and disadvantaged children. We utilize a combination of volunteer dentists and a few small grants to provide services to over 25,000 mid-state families each year.

That's it! That's all most people will care about in your *how* and *what.* You may think your internal processes are too complex to be summed up in a sentence or two. You are correct, but look at this sentence:

At GEICO a fifteen-minute call could save you fifteen percent or more on your car insurance.

Do you think GEICO's internal processes are complex? Of course. Is it possible GEICO has a considerably more complicated business than yours? Most likely. So why do they persist in saying this simple line? Because GEICO understands the audience is not interested in the internal workings of their company. Tell us their *how* and *what* but keep it as simple as possible.

Connect to Purpose Story

A *Connect to Purpose Story* is the *result* of your organization living their *why*. Because you believe everyone deserves primary dental care, here is a story of a real person whose life was improved. Your organization's *why* has helped correct painful dental problems, which would have negatively impacted that patient's life. Your *Connect to Purpose Story* is told to illustrate actual benefits received as a result of your organization living their why.

A *Connect to Purpose Story* might sound like this:

(Start with your *why*)

> At Ceranos Learning Academy we believe every child can learn, including those who struggle in the traditional learning environment.

(Move into your *how and what*)
> That's why we have developed a complex system of assessment tools that reveal exactly how your child learns. We can instruct them in the method best for them, not the best method for the school.

(Finish with your *Connect to Purpose Story*)
> David was our student a few years ago. His mother was heartbroken because she knew her son was smart, but he struggled with individual teachers and subjects. During the assessments, we saw David had a tremendous need for autonomy and discovery. Once our teachers started asking David questions instead of giving him answers, he progressed quickly. He went on to complete four years of high school, and now he is studying engineering at Georgia Tech.

Connect to Purpose Stories are everywhere, but you have to train yourself and your staff to recognize and harvest them. At a team meeting, you might say, "We are looking for real stories about real people whose lives have been made better because of what we do." Then give them a few examples of Connect to Purpose Stories. You'll be surprised at how many personal stories your staff already knows, and how quick they are to share new stories as they happen.

Once you start collecting Connect to Purpose stories, you may find a journal is an efficient way to record them. Margaret shared a few stories from her "Purpose Journal" recently. Once she started looking for them, she was able to see many occasions where "good work" within her organization was an opportunity to connect her *why, how* and *what* to these real-life situations.

"This I Believe" formula

We need to have a *mean*ingful conversation. Speaking about the weather, the latest sports scores or mindless trivia does not captivate any audience. If you want to move people, to change people, to make a difference in the lives of other people, you need to say something important to them in your limited time in the spotlight.

A formula we call "This I believe" allows you to have that critical conversation.

Beginning in 1951 radio pioneer, Edward R. Murrow asked everyday Americans about their most fundamental beliefs. The ensuing essays became a part of an NPR radio program and later two books (Picadoor, 2006). Each article is less than 500 words but contains deep and personally meaningful messages.

Being an avid reader, I love to give books away as gifts. I have given away more *"This I Believe"* books than any other single title. *"This I Believe,"* to me, is the formula for having a conversation that matters. In our one-on-one classes, we teach strategies following this formula that has dramatically changed the way our clients speak.

The formula begins with choosing a *deeply held belief* that is personally meaningful to you. This formula takes some work. The method does not work if you want as your subject something everyday, trivial, or predictable.

Here are some examples from *"This I Believe:"*

- I believe that freedom is contagious. *Harold Kongju Koh*
- I believe in the power of the unknown. I believe that a sense of the unknown

propels us in all of our creative activities, from science to art. *Alan Lightman*
- Jazz is the sound of God laughing, and I believe in it. *Colleen Shaddok*
- I believe listening is powerful medicine. *Alicia Conill*
- I believe in America, and I believe in our people. *Colin Powell*

This formula takes some soul-searching and frankly some soul bearing. Most of the time we try to shield our deepest beliefs and repackage them in more widely acceptable words before sharing them with others. Saying out loud to others something meaningful from the depths of our being is hard, but the connection we make with others when we do is more than worth it.

Step one: say something meaningful.

What is the boldest possible statement you can make? A friend and client responded with, "I believe in the rule of law. I believe we get it right most of the time. I believe most judges and juries and attorneys work feverishly to get it right." Another client begins her presentation with, "We are hurtling out of the mean-spirited darkness of the past into a bright future that will be more generous, kind and caring than at any time in history."

Boldness has power. Building a great speech based on a bold statement is easy. A weak statement does not inspire, and often the words are hard to find based on a tepid opening statement. If you see yourself stuck, revisit your opening *This I Believe* statement and make sure it is fearless.

However, what if someone disagrees with us? That's good. Adult learners often argue as part of the learning process. We can tell an engaged audience by the number of opposing arguments we get, and engagement is fundamental to all communication.

Your opening statement does not need to include the phrase, "This I believe." A bolder way to begin may be to say it as if it is true. "Diversity is America's greatest strength" is stronger than "I believe diversity is America's greatest strength." You might find it's even better to start with a story that demonstrates what you are talking about and save your "This I believe" statement until later paragraphs.
For instance:

> "When I was a young boy I watched a homeless man with a dog beg at a street

corner. A car pulled up and handed the man a fast food bag. The homeless man opened the bag and fed most of the food to the dog. Only after the dog ate did the homeless man feed himself.

When people ask me why I believe the world is getting better, I tell them we live in a world where often the dog eats first."

Step two: build a couple of supporting statements.

My "I believe" statement:

"I believe the world is getting better."

Supporting statements
- Violent crime in the US dropped 48% between 1993 and 2016.
- High school cigarette smoking has declined from 10.7% in 1991 to 1.8% last year.
- Global death rates from war have declined from 22 per 100,000 people to 3.

Step three: admit and deal with opposing arguments.

> *Many people would disagree. Their brains poisoned by endless cable news programs, they tend to believe we are much worse off now than before. However, the facts do not back that up. In virtually every statistically significant measurement we are safer, live longer and better, and care about each other in ways our ancestors never dreamed.*

If you choose a sufficiently bold statement, there will be people who do not agree with you. Acknowledging those arguments and dealing with them is vital to the effectiveness of your presentation.

I would caution you not to delve into a *straw man* argument. The 'straw man' is a restatement of the opposing argument in such a way as to make it easily defeated, but not truthful. In the example above if you said,

> *Some people would have you believe the world is so violent today that murders and violence happen on every street corner without so much as the public notice.*

No one believes that. The more thoughtful people in your audience will dismiss this argument and likely everything else you say.

Step four: expound on the impact your premise will have if true.

> Continuing declines in violent crime mean fewer police and prisons. The absence of war would mean military contractors could focus on infrastructure projects. Children that never smoke cigarettes are exposed to fewer causes of cancer, which would significantly cut our future healthcare costs.

Step five: conclude with a summation statement.

A summation statement will be similar to your "This I believe" statement with which you began. However, if anything, this is more of a personal creed or vision statement rather than a premise.

> Yes indeed, the world is getting better. This is not just a radical idea from a lone crackpot. All the available evidence supports this. This is science. This is statistics. This is true.

> Because this is true, we need to begin to reject the naysayers and fear mongers who would have us cower in our homes and fear

our neighbors and those who do not look like us or believe the way we do.

So that's it. We have worked through this formula with quite a few speakers. Every time they end up with a moving and inspirational presentation. The method has worked for architects and attorneys, school children and chefs, CEOs and supervisors, and every time it has allowed the speaker to create a meaningful conversation. Try it and let us know how it works for you.

Step Four
Storytelling Basics

People won't forget your story or anecdote

Speaking is indeed synonymous with storytelling. Since the beginning of human speech, we've used stories to pass on information and make our points. Roman and Greek mythological stories were passed down through the generations to help the people understand their relationships with their gods. Aesop's Fables taught--and still do teach-- principles of behavior that guide society. At a time when people could not read, stories were the critical methods for transferring cultural knowledge. Today, however, theater, music, poetry, dance, novels, short stories, visual arts, movies, television and audio books are the variety of methods we use. They are merely stories told in different forms. We learn quicker from accounts than any other type of communication. We remember longer what we encounter in stories. We experience more in-depth and more thoroughly the information we receive in stories.

If you want to make your point memorable for a long time, tell it regarding a story.

> *Gandhi was well known for his selflessness and care for all of humanity. Traveling once by train, his sandal slipped beneath a gap in the walkway. Gandhi quickly took off his remaining sandal and threw it also beneath the gap. Asked why, Gandhi said, "Should a poor person find only one sandal, they would have no use, but finding two would be wonderful."*

Remember we do not tell stories to entertain; we tell stories to educate and elevate our audience. The Gandhi story seems full of wisdom, but it is up to you to connect it to your content.

> *Like Gandhi, if we create this new process but fail to implement the training, it is like the poor person finding only one sandal.*

We learn from stories
Before the printed word, stories were essential to the sharing of knowledge. Indeed, our earliest

ancestors might have never started this amazing progress to what we are today had it not been for their ability to convey information through language. Their stories pushed each new generation forward with the accumulated knowledge of all previous ages. Using language to tell and learn from stories was the marker separating Homo sapiens from the rest. As Ian Leslie says in his book, *Curious*:

> *"About sixty thousand years ago, a small population of humans journeyed out of Africa and struck out for the unknown.*
>
> *"Our ancestors lived by the sea, learned to fish and traveled to cold climates and learned to adapt. Our closest relatives, the apes, never left the forest, but humans figured out how to fish and hunt and live in diverse environments because they have one remarkable skill, the ability to communicate complex stories across generations."*

Universally, we tell stories, all cultures, all places, all times. Hansel and Gretel, Adam and Eve, David and Goliath, Romeo and Juliet. Stories are the way we understand the world and how we pass that knowledge to others.

I do not have to touch the stove to know it's hot. Someone else has already done that and warned us through their stories. The young child learns how to behave through examples conveyed in stories. Jesus was asked why he told parables and he responded, "This is why I speak to them in parables, because seeing they do not see, and hearing they do not hear, nor do they understand (Matthew 13:13). When you have a complex subject like salvation or grace, and you're trying to teach it to shepherds and fishermen, a good story goes a long way.

Somehow in the business world, we forget this valuable lesson. We load up our presentation with bullet points, pie charts and elaborate details that leave our audience lost and disinterested. At the end of our seemingly well-crafted speech, our audience leaves the room without one key takeaway. There is no story to hang those key points on.

Tell stories to communicate your point

Your stories serve one purpose: to communicate a point to the audience. We do not tell stories to tell stories. Start with what you think you need to communicate, and then find a way to communicate that through a story. Ask yourself, what *point* am I trying to make? Then communicate that point by establishing a connection with it and a story that helps your audience remember it.

Stories should be as short as possible

You may have heard the saying, "If you ask him what time it is, he will tell you how the watch was made." A story works when it is as brief as possible but still long enough to do the job. Try trimming it shorter and shorter. If any detail is not necessary for the story to work, kick it out. Get others you trust to listen to the story and ask them if the story is too long.

Tell your own story

For many of us, the most powerful thing we can share with others is our own story. Look back at my story about being voted "Quietest." You learned about my struggle, my weaknesses, my determination and my eventual success. You probably have your own story of struggle and redemption. Look for it; listen to it, and practice sharing it so that it becomes a useful tool for you.

We build stories like this: A likable protagonist wants something intensely. They go out to get it, but something blocks their way. Eventually, they find a way to overcome the obstacle and get the thing they desired, but most importantly they become a different person than who they were when they started the journey.

Tell your story in present tense

Present tense means you speak about things as though they are happening now, not in the past.

> "Amelia Earhart has a problem. Try as she might, she cannot locate the island where she is to refuel. She is not aware the direction finder on the island has a dead battery. She doesn't know her plane has been outfitted with the wrong type of antennae. Earhart does not know the flight patterns given to her are miscalculated. What she does know is she is running low on fuel and is a long way from her next stop."

Present tense gives greater tension to a story than past tense. Present tense feels real and vital.

Invite your audience in

Chances are good your audience is not thinking, "Oh, boy, I wonder when she is going to tell me a story?" They are lost in their mental world. So how do you get them to begin to go with you on this journey? Invite them in. Ask them a question that will get their attention and connect with your story. Something like:

> 1. Have you ever been angry? Really angry? Like you cannot even make words you are so angry?
>
> 2. Remember those Pop Rocks? That carbonated candy that kind of exploded in your mouth? Did you have those growing up?
>
> 3. We've all had times when we were afraid, haven't we? Think back on a time when you were honestly afraid of something.

Now you've got them thinking and feeling, and you've primed them for your story. Give your audience a few seconds to thoughtfully reminisce about that feeling, and then move into your story.

> When I was little, I was afraid of many things but more than anything I was terrified of the dark. How about you? Were you ever terrified of something? Can you remember being little; lying in bed and being so incredibly afraid you cannot even

> move because of your fear? (Pause and let them remember how it felt)
>
> Doctors call it 'terror paralysis,' and we all have it, but for James Mentle it controls his life. When he fears something, he becomes catatonic.

Invite your audience to live your story with you

What would they see if they were there? What sounds would they hear? What smells would they smell? What would they feel if they were in your story? A few well-placed cues can help your audience see what you see and hear what you hear.

> "It's March 16th, 2002, my birthday, and I am sitting in my brand new, midnight blue Mazda Miata. Imagine sitting with me. You feel that supple Italian leather seat? You feel the spring breeze blow through your hair? On the radio, we hear Al Jarreau. Around us, we smell the honeysuckle in full bloom."

By describing what we see, hear, smell and feel you can quickly take your audience into the story and let them live it as if they were there. Ask these questions about your audience:

>What would *they see* if they were there?
>What would *they feel* if they were there?
>What would *they smell* if they were there?
>What would *they hear* if they were there?

The story setup above takes only a few seconds, but you will be able to pull your audience into your story quickly by using these cues.

Don't announce your story, begin it

Our audiences do not need all the transitions. Inexperienced speakers think they have to announce they are going to tell a story, but there is no need. "Let me tell you a story about when I was in Pakistan." Don't. Instead, begin. "October 9th, 2011, I am stranded at the Sindhri Airport in Sindhri, Pakistan." Don't build up to it and do not announce it. Launch with both feet straight into your story.

Forget about transition phrases

Most transitions are unnecessary. "If we could go back a bit..." or "Now let's talk about patient data."

There is no need. From a lifetime of watching TV and movies, we've all gotten accustomed to switching subjects in lightning speeds. Our protagonist meets a girl on a train in Boston, and almost immediately we cut to his father's funeral in Sri Lanka. As the casket descends into the grave, we hear a plane landing and the airport announcer, "For passengers arriving at Charles De Gaulle airport, please remember to keep your bags with you at all times." The filmmakers have removed all of the setups and build-ups and announcements. We live in a cut/cut/cut world, and our speaking style needs to reflect that.

Change the scene rapidly and without notice

One might think changing scenes every few minutes would be disconcerting, but it is not. What Hollywood has figured out is that to keep people on the edge of their seats, they need to change the scene rapidly and without warning. That's good advice to us as speakers.

Let's pace out our presentation like we would if we worked for Paramount.

> Scene one: Protagonist CEO is cheered as he becomes youngest ever CEO in the one hundred and ten-year history of this respected health system.

> Cut to:
> Scene two: Late night as CEO and CFO flip through spreadsheet after spreadsheet. CEO says: "This is bad." CFO: "Told you."
> Cut to:
> Scene three: Rain falls as solitary runner stops in the middle of a deserted four-way stop. He looks first left and then right. Close up on his face reveals he is our CEO.
>
> Cut to:
> Scene four: Break room fills with employees finding their seats. At the front of the room is the CEO, no tie, sleeves rolled up, looking like he has not slept. "I debated telling you this," he says as his voice trails off, "but you need to know. This hospital is broke, and without a dramatic and immediate infusion of cash we face...bankruptcy."

This story has action, suspense, and passion. How do we do this in a speech?

> "January 18, 2010, was the best day of my life. At the age of thirty-two, I became the youngest CEO of Avalex Memorial Health System. I was ecstatic.

Once the excitement and congratulations died down, our CFO and I dug into the numbers. It was terrible, really, really bad. Avalex...is...broke.

My first CEO job was about to be my last, and I did what I always do when my mind is swirling. I went out for a long run. Somewhere along Marcos Road where it intersects with the old highway 45, I stopped. I watched the rainfall, and I pondered my next move. To my left was avoidance. I could continue to cover up the problem while I furiously looked for another job. Ahead was denial. I could merely deny there was a problem until someone came and locked the door. To the right...well, that was you.

Many of you have put your heart and soul into Avalex. Many of you had parents or grandparents who worked here. This tragedy isn't my tragedy; this is our tragedy. I decided to come clean, and that is why I am here in front of you. I have no easy answers, and even if we do everything right, we may still have to close the doors. What we face is not easy, but this is a challenge we will face together."

Build tension with a puzzle

People love to solve puzzles. Whether it's crossword puzzles or sudoku, humans spend an enormous amount of time with puzzles. Why, then, would we rob our audience of that enjoyment? Too often we see presentations that begin with the answer, then go on to illustrate the steps taken to get to that answer. We format our talk like this:

1. The teen had Cohn's Disease.
2. We did not know so we tried other things.
3. None of those worked until we discovered it was Cohn's.

How much more interesting it would be if we started with the puzzle and let the audience try to figure it out along the way, like this:

1. The teen appeared to have a cardiac event.
2. We tested and could not find the defect.
3. Then we thought maybe it was cancer.
4. When that turned out not to be the case we tried some additional tests.

5. Finally, we determined it was Cohn's Disease.

Much of the work of healthcare is solving puzzles. A patient presents with a set of symptoms. The care team goes through a system of diagnostics to try to determine the cause. Time passes, and one by one the care team dismisses possible causes until finally a correct diagnosis is determined. Proper treatment then ensues, and the patient gets better.

It is this puzzle/solution process that makes the TV show "House" so compelling. Imagine if the show began with the correct diagnosis and then the search came after. Can you imagine how uninteresting a program like that would be?

Step Five
Rules of Engagement

Speaking success is business success

Think about it; we almost never see a business leader who isn't also an accomplished speaker. Whether we are talking about Steve Jobs or Sir Richard Branson, Sheryl Sandberg or Jeff Bezos, the great leaders, the ones that inspire us, are almost always great speakers.

In 2004 at the Democratic National Convention a young man stood on stage and spoke twenty-two hundred words, for some seventeen minutes, and changed the course of history. The day before no one had ever heard of Barack Obama; the day after no one could ever forget him. My point is not about politics, but about you and your ability to change your world through your speaking skills.

Many years ago, Carnegie Institute of Technology released a study that said eighty-five percent of your success in the next five years has to do with your ability to speak and communicate your ideas. Eighty-five percent. That's more than the boost from your degree, more than your years in the industry. That's more than your connections. Hard to believe, but eighty-five percent *of your success in the next five years* is dependent on your ability to speak well and communicate your ideas effectively. Typically, if you or I want to improve our worth in the marketplace, we would get an advanced degree such as an MBA or a Ph.D. However, how long would that take and how much would it cost? Bloomberg Money puts the cost of an MBA at $296,000. The Carnegie study contends that eighty-five percent of your success depends on your ability to speak and communicate your ideas well. So which investment is worth your time and money?

Soft skills versus hard skills
Hard skills are what most of us learn in school: math, science, accounting, programming, and biology. By contrast, soft skills include communication, teamwork, management, coaching, and presenting. Hard skills require IQ, and soft skills require EQ or emotional intelligence. As we look ahead at the future of work, tasks requiring hard skills can be automated, but at least for now soft skills still need a human.

The workplace is undergoing seismic changes
Today, well-respected fields involving hard skills are increasingly using artificial intelligence. Robots *are* coming for our jobs. The Pew Research Center estimates thirty-eight percent of all current jobs will disappear in the next fifteen years. Just during the time, the nation has spent arguing about the Keystone Oil Pipeline, solar power has become cheaper than gas. Keystone may no longer make sense. Self-driving trucks are here. Australia uses huge self-driving trucks in their mining industry twenty-four hours a day, nights, weekends, and holidays, with no breaks. No time off for a Foster's and a vegemite sandwich, mate!

Robots in my field?
Surely that won't happen to you and me, will it? I remember while in college I came across my first ATM in downtown Murfreesboro, Tennessee. I thought it was the dumbest thing I had ever seen. A machine to take deposits and dispense cash? How ridiculous. I wanted a real person on the other side of the counter when taking care of my money. Shortly after, in 1977, Citibank took a gamble and spent almost one hundred million dollars installing ATMs all over New York City. The following January there was a blizzard that

closed down the city. Only the people who were lucky enough to be Citibank customers had access to their money via ATMs. Within five years ATMs spread to almost every corner of the world.

Before 1977, we never thought banks would be affected by automation. However, how long has it been since you have been inside a bank? Today, most of us would gladly pay the three-dollar ATM fee to avoid having to park and wait in line to talk to someone at the counter. So, will the automation that happened in banking affect you and your job? Will you wake up one day to discover you are an expert in the hard skills of business that no longer exist?

Here's the good news
The soft skills of speaking effectively to any audience, that is, *Public Speaking,* can be learned with relative ease and will always be in demand. During this training, you will learn how to shape your message in such a way that your audience initially attends and stays engaged to the very end. You will learn how to organize and deliver your message so that your audience hears what you intend them to understand. I have worked with clients both through one-on-one private coaching and within a classroom setting. I have seen people who start out rough---very rough--

and four weeks later are exhibiting a high level of speaking skill. It takes dedication and practice, but if you apply your focused attention you, too, can become a skilled presenter.

The Halo Effect
The Halo Effect suggests that when you are good at something we can see, we assume you are also probably good at things we cannot see. For instance, if you are a skilled presenter with clear ideas, carefully chosen words, vibrant examples, and engaging delivery, we can assume you are probably also good at other things, like being an effective leader, a solid fiscal manager, or a devoted employee.

The Halo Effect was initially described in a study at the University of Minnesota by Dion, Berscheid & Walster (1972). Sixty students were shown pictures of three individuals and asked to predict the person on twenty-seven different traits, including such as altruism, conventionality, self-assertiveness, stability, emotionality, trustworthiness, extraversion, kindness, and sexual promiscuity. Ahead of time, the photos had been selected as examples of an attractive person, an average person, and an unattractive person. The beautiful person (a trait we can see) was guessed to have many more positive characteristics (traits we cannot see) than the unattractive person.

Is this fair? No, but you can use this to your advantage. By becoming a skilled speaker, your value within the organization will go up as the audience assumes you have other positive traits as well. I know anecdotally that when I speak on stage, people often believe I am smarter than I am.

You must be engaging
When we talk about speaking situations, we typically think of a presenter at a conference, but in reality, we all use what speaking skills we have on a daily basis. The teacher in a classroom, the department head or supervisor within an organization, the chair of business or civic committee, the committee members themselves, the employees dealing with the public, whatever the role, we most frequently use speech to communicate our message. Sometimes the communication is short and direct, and the audience is eager to hear what the speaker has to say. More often, though, the communication is more detailed and lengthy, and the audience may be distracted, sleepy, or otherwise disinterested.

Teachers know the challenge of maintaining student attention, as do skilled preachers at lengthy Sunday sermons, and executives reporting dry details of a business. It's true; extenuating circumstances can make it harder to engage an audience (after lunch, the last session of the day, room too hot or cold, outside noises), but the speaker is still responsible for capturing and keeping that audience engaged. If you are the speaker and your audience is not interested in what you are saying for whatever reason, they will check out, lean back, pull out their phones and start making a shopping list. On occasion conference speakers see audience members walk out of their presentation. *Engagement is our first responsibility. Without engagement, nothing else matters.*

I have worked in television for thirty-five years. In TV we are keenly aware that our audience is fickle. We huddle around a spreadsheet of numbers each morning to see how we did with our audience the night before. In five-minute increments, we see people tune in, look around, then bug out. Those TV viewers have a remote control that gives them one hundred fifty other options in a tenth of a second if we are not marvelously engaging. We lived for engagement. We died by engagement. It was like a drug for us. At one time if our five o'clock news rating was doing well and rose from a 4.4 to a 4.5, our station looked to make a million-dollar profit. When engagement is worth one million dollars, you pay attention.

My speaker training includes many of the techniques I have learned in the television industry making commercials. Over the years I have put more than ten thousand people on camera. Each time I instructed the speaker on what to say, how to say it, what to do with their hands, what clothes work best, where to stand and when to move. An engaging TV commercial can propel a small business ahead, and a boring ad can sink a small business. I took my job seriously, and I take the responsibility of public speaking seriously as well.

A few years ago, I began video work for Quint Studer and his team at the Studer Group. There I worked with accomplished speakers like Quint and ten other world-class speakers like him.

I also came to know the subject matter experts who shared their stories to improve healthcare around the world. Often these experts were amateurs in public speaking, and my job was to help them tell a compelling story.

If you speak to an audience of one hundred and fifty people for one hour, and on average each audience member earns a salary of $50 an hour, you've just blown through $7,500 of their time. Is the content you provide worth $7,500? It better be. We cheat our audience when we show up at a $7,500 event and give a $500 speech.

Audiences ask, "What's in this for me?"
When you spend time with some of the very best speakers in the field as well as with amateurs, it quickly becomes clear who speaks well and who does not. For each of these speakers, the paramount focus is on getting the audience engaged and keeping them engaged.

If you study the subject of effective public speaking as much as I have, you will encounter many terrible ideas that claim to enhance your speaking abilities. One of the most egregious is, *picture your audience naked.* The level of absurdity contained in that statement is alarming. Instead, imagine your audience with this phrase emblazoned on their foreheads: *What's in this for me?*

One of our most precious commodities is our attention. We live in a world that screams for attention all the time. TV, newspapers, movies, iPods and cell phones shout headlines or buzz and vibrate with a dizzying array of attention-seeking strategies. Your audience is making a bet that your presentation is worth the few minutes of their limited attention. From the time they read the topic of your presentation in the program to the moment they leave your presentation, they are asking themselves: *What am I going to get out of this talk?*

Your failure to answer this question can fatally spoil your presentation. Answer it quickly and explain it often. Your audience is looking for ways to apply this information to their lives, but also looking for ways to dismiss your information, saying in essence, *this isn't something I need to listen to*. Each member of your audience wants to be in the know and hopes your presentation will:

- Make me smarter
- Keep my family and me safe
- Help my career
- Entertain me
- Help me save or make money
- Inspire me
- Make me part of something important.

There are dozens of more reasons, but keep in mind that your audience is hungry for information that can improve their lives. Get there quickly and *stay there*. If you find yourself disconnected from the audience's *"What's in it for me?"* question, your speech will feel flat, and your audience will leave feeling cheated.

The Quietest
In 1976 I was mad at the world and just "over it." My family had moved for the millionth time and landed in the middle of nowhere, in some backward, rural community with more cows than people. It is not that we *wanted* to move; it is just that we were poor. We would move into a new neighborhood, get behind on rent and then get evicted by the landlord. Wash, rinse, and repeat.

It was never easy to go to a new school and try to make new friends, so this time I just gave up. I did not think I would like this town or the people, so I did not try. I figured I would be out of school in a few years and I did not want or need any of those people to be my friends. Fast-forward a couple of years, and my yearbook voted me, "Quietest." That's right. While the rest of my world was being voted "Best Looking," "Most Athletic," or "Most Likely to Succeed," I was voted "Quietest." In my view, that was quite the opposite of "Most Likely to Succeed."

At first, I chose not to talk in school because I did not *want* to, but by the time the yearbook came out, I did not speak to anyone *because I did not know how to.* Social skills are like muscles; if you don't use them, they atrophy. My reluctance to engage with other students blunted my ability. So, I was miserable. Being "Quietest" meant getting none of the good things out of life. I did not get good grades because I was afraid to raise my hand in class. I did not get the girl because I could not flirt and ask her out. I did not get the job because I needed to walk in somewhere to inquire.

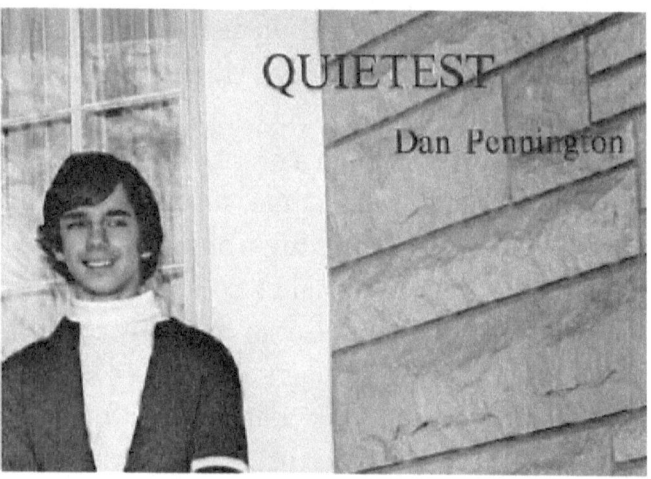

So how do you get to be *Quiet*? The same way someone runs a marathon. A little at a time. No one runs twenty-six miles on day one. You get there a tiny bit at a time. If you do not raise your hand today, it becomes much more difficult tomorrow. If you sit by yourself quietly at lunch, the thought of inviting yourself to someone else's table seems hugely daunting. My original obstinacy had led me to a crippling shyness.

How did I solve my problem? I have always been an avid reader. I went to my school library and read books on psychology. After all, I thought, if I can figure out people, I can figure out how to get out of this self-induced shyness. I read every book in that library related to sociology or psychology. The librarian noticed my interest and asked the janitor to show me a back room that was piled high with out-of-circulation textbooks.

"Take 'em," he said. "Take as many as you want." From there I loaded up armfuls of more psychology books that later covered my desk at home.

So then, there it was. A simple quote:

> "The 'self-image' is the key to human personality and human behavior. Change the self-image, and you change the personality and the behavior."
>
> Maxwell Maltz

None of us can ever go beyond our self-image. There I was, trapped with the self-image of a shy person, and that image was a chain holding me back. Have you ever seen a dog in someone's backyard on a chain? The dog cuts a semicircle out of the grass at the furthest point the chain allows him to travel. Want a different life? You need a longer chain, or even better, no chain at all.

Over time I forced myself to do things a shy person would never do. I tried out for a minor role in a stage play. I worked my way onto the debate team. However, most importantly, I changed the way I talked to myself about myself.

I tell you this story because so often students in my class will say; "This is easy for you, Daniel because you are so outgoing. Me? Well...I'm just shy." I tell them, "Listen, sister, I've got you beat. I won an *award* for being shy!"
Get outside of your comfort zone

Look at any successful person, and one thing is likely true about them. They have become *comfortable* with being *uncomfortable*. You may have seen this diagram before:

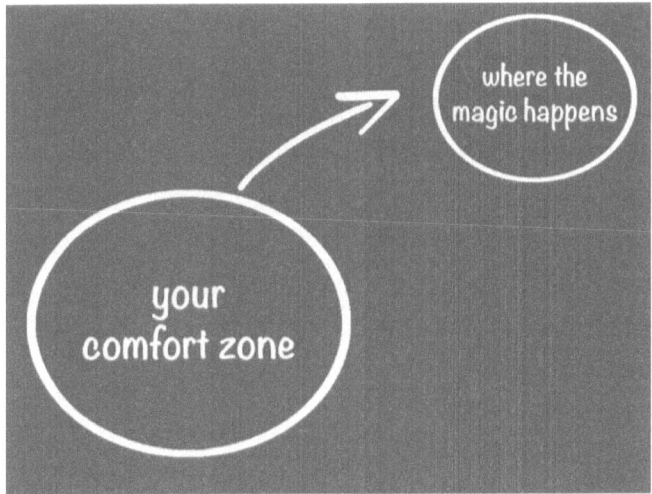

If any of us is going to grow and develop at all, we have to get comfortable with being uncomfortable. Being at the front of the room is challenging. What if people do not like you? What if they do not laugh at your humor or you forget your place in the presentation? That's uncomfortable. However, here is a fundamental truth: your audience *wants* you to succeed. Always remember others are eager for you to do well.

By now I have taught enough speaking classes and worked with enough individual clients to see a predictable pattern arise when people first move out of their comfort zone. Fear and DIScomfort loom large, so I have developed several strategies to help people gradually expand their boundaries.

Overcoming jitters

I break the six-person team in half, with three of them instructed to stand in front of the room as "presenters" and the other three as the audience. The presenters are to do nothing, stand there. We stare at them; they stare at us. At first, our presenters think this is funny. Then they get nervous; they fidget, look at the floor. We can tell they are uncomfortable. I ask them how it feels, and they emphatically say, "Awful!"

The Police Interrogation Exercise

Next, I give them a task. I tell them to pretend that those of us in the audience go missing *just minutes* after this class. Police come in and question them about us. What color hair does he have? How tall is she? What blouse is she wearing? Jewelry? What age would you guess? Thin? Muscular? Heavy? I ask our presenters to try to remember every detail, so they can recount it correctly later. When I use this exercise, a fantastic thing happens at this point. Our presenters no longer look nervous. As soon as they stop focusing on themselves and they put their entire focus on the audience their nerves calm down.

Your glasses are on backward
When we are nervous about being up in front of people, it is because we have our glasses on backward. We buy glasses to see better what is *out there.* However, we get self-conscious when our focus is *in here,* on ourselves. By doing the Police Interrogation Exercise, we can refocus our attention away from us and out onto everyone else.

You can try this yourself without being in a class. Go to your local big box retailer and pretend everyone you meet goes missing, and you have to describe him or her later. How does the greeter look? Hair color? Eye color? You are not paying close enough attention to others unless you can recall their eye color later.

Go into the shoe section and ask a question, but rather than paying attention to the answer, study the salesperson. How tall is she? What age would you guess? What color is her blouse? Does she have a bit of an accent? Repeat this in each section of the store. Is the pharmacist in his fifties? Sixties, maybe? Try again in the deli and produce. Start with one question to get them to stop and talk, and then remember as many details about them as possible.

Once you have done this a few times, you get much better at it. You will begin to notice things no one else does. When you ask the deli guy if his accent is from Philadelphia, he will be thrilled that you noticed, and you may end up with a couple of extra croissants in your order.

Humans have a universal yearning to be noticed, to matter to someone. When we pay close attention to them, they blossom. Joe Girard sold more cars than any other salesman in history. In fact, he sold more than thirteen thousand vehicles in the fourteen years of doing business. How did he do it? In part by sending out a greeting card to every client he ever had, every single month! That meant every month he sent out thirteen thousand cards, and each card had a straightforward sentiment on it, "Happy New Year, I like you, Joe Girard." Every month thirteen thousand people felt great because Joe Girard made it clear he likes them.

Get to know your audience first
When you are talking to a group, you seldom run in the door and immediately begin speaking. There is often a settling period where people get

coffee during a brief break between presentations. Before it is your time to talk, do the Police Lineup Exercise with the folks who will be in your audience. Notice them, focusing entirely on them. Then when you step on stage, make it clear that you like them by paying close attention to them and not yourself.

> *"Stewart was telling me before I got on stage how much this group has grown."* Stewart is thrilled you noticed him.
> *"Jamie, this probably ties into some of your charity work, doesn't it?"* Jamie is thrilled you listened.

Coping with nerves

The first and most important tip I can share with you is to know and completely understand your subject. As we train people, we can see in their faces as they struggle to remember their next words and sentences. No person is ever confident who is also struggling to retain content. Know, understand, and comprehend your material. If you and I were called on to explain algebraic equations, we would hem and haw all of our way through it. If, however, we were asked to describe why we love someone we would do it without a problem. The more immersed in the subject, the smoother the delivery.

Next step is to tell a story. Stories usually have a predictable set of components: an open and close, a protagonist and antagonist, tension and resolution. Because we are familiar with the structure of a story we usually don't struggle with knowing what comes next.

Ask for feedback from someone you trust. The more you refine and clarify your presentation based on reliable feedback the more confident you'll be in the delivery. Ask for specifics. Did this last too long? Were you able to follow this story? Did my examples make everything clear? What questions are you left with? Does this feel fresh or is it something you feel like you've heard before?

Place all of your focus on your audience. Watch their faces. Are they nodding? Smiling? Do they look confused or bored? If you put all of your attention on your audience, you won't have time to focus on your nerves.

Stages of training
As you go through this training process, you will likely experience a predictable set of steps.

The honeymoon period. At the outset, students almost always have a great deal of enthusiasm for the training and have visions of being a captivating speaker.

Reality sets in. After the initial excitement comes the shock of realizing how difficult giving an excellent presentation can be. Participants become dismayed by their lack of skills and often wonder if they will ever become the effective speakers they desire to be.

Dark times. This is the time when the real work begins the fun wears off, and the student gets into the hard work. Progress comes more slowly, and it feels like many false starts and dead ends. This step can be an especially tough time for some.

Breakthrough success. As with learning any new skill participants will find renewed excitement as they begin to encounter mastery. The first few times students use the new techniques and achieve positive results can be energizing. As they practice and eventually master these new skills their confidence increases.

It's going to happen

These things will happen when you are learning to become a better speaker:

1. Your humor will fall short.
2. The audience will seem confused.
3. A technical failure will occur.
4. You will lose your place.
5. Someone's cell phone will go off.
6. Someone in the audience will look bored or sleepy.
7. An emergency will happen.

However, in any of these instances, it is not the end of the world. You can overcome them.

Use the If/Then strategy

If we know that at some point negative things are going to happen, we can strategize beforehand how we would deal with them when they do occur. The U.S. Army Special Forces take time before each mission to go through every possible mistake that *could happen* and develop a strategy for what to do next. I call them if/then strategy AR-DR, or:

Acknowledge, Reframe, Defuse, Resume

Prepare your strategies in advance, so *if* things happen, *then* you will know what to do and be ready to respond.

Acknowledge

Make your audience aware of what is happening and be clear you know what is happening as well. People in the back of the room or seated further away may not be aware of a disturbance and, therefore, wonder why some audience members are reacting as they are.

Reframe

It is up to you to role model how the rest of the room is going to feel about this. If you become upset, they likely will also. Instead, take a professional stance and expect your audience to do the same.

Defuse

When the unexpected happens, we feel the tension. Defusing the tension allows both you and the audience to get back to your message.

Resume

Only after you've done these three, (Acknowledge, Reframe, and Defuse) should you move on. However, do not rush it if the interruption was significant, for example, a fire alarm. It may take the audience some time to calm down enough to proceed.

Here are some scenarios:
A cell phone goes off, and the audience member answers it while exiting the room

> *Acknowledge*
> "For those of you in the back, let me tell you what just happened. A person up front got a phone call that he needed to answer before going out in the hall."
>
> *Reframe*
> "We all have phones, and we never know when we must answer that important call. Let's hope they are closing the big deal right now. No sweat. It happens."
>
> *Defuse*
> "However, the rule is, if you answer your phone during the session you have to buy doughnuts...for everyone! So, when they get back, we'll take a moment to get everyone's order. Okay? Chocolate iced glazed with sprinkles for me."
>
> *Resume*
> "So, while we wait for doughnuts, I think we can go on with the message. Are you with me?"

A waiter drops an entire tray of dishes.

Acknowledge
"For those of you who are up front, someone in the wait staff just dropped a tray of dishes."

Reframe
"I hope he is all right. Can we get someone to check? The staff here has been wonderful, and that can happen to anyone."

Defuse
"You know, gravity is not just a good idea...it's the law."

Resume
"As they get that picked up I would like to continue with this thought. Would that be okay? Are we not too distracted to listen? Are you with me? Great, let's move on."

Memorizing is hard work

At this point in our training, my clients look at me with wide-open eyes and almost scream, "This is hard work!" Somewhere along the way, they had come to believe an excellent presentation could be created and delivered without tremendous effort. I am sorry to say this is not true. Effective communication requires an enormous amount of time and effort, and there is no way to shortchange that.

With that, we come to what is perhaps the most tedious part of the process, or at least it is for me, memorization. The question always arises, do I entirely write out the presentation and memorize it word for word, or do I jot down a handful of bullet points and deliver from those? The best answer may depend on you, but most of us use a combination of both.

Writing your presentation out long form allows you to wordsmith it a bit. You remove unnecessary words and phrases and find tighter, more effective ways to say things. My friend Shannon mentioned in her presentation, "That's a grim fact that has allowed generational poverty to take hold of some neighborhoods by the throat, keeping the parents and children who live their hostage." Isn't that a beautiful use of language? I do not think anyone could have phrased that so correctly without having written it out previously.

A shorter presentation, say twenty to thirty minutes, is relatively easy for most of us to type up. If you're not a great typist, Google.docs has a helpful feature used by many. You speak, and it types the words out, similar to texting by talking rather than typing your message. Most users rate it as reasonably accurate. Longer presentations say an hour or more can be challenging to write out completely. I still do this for my talks, but I'm a reasonably proficient typist.

We then recommend you rehearse directly from your complete script, reading it word for word until you've almost committed it to memory. It will likely take dozens of repetitions until you master it. You can also record it on your phone and play it back over and over again.

Stand up and move around while you are memorizing. Research shows that standing up aids memorization. Read it all out loud, not silently. Get your mouth and tongue used to the words and phrases. At this time rework anything challenging to say. Spoken speech and written speech are dramatically different. In writing we can understand and follow complex sentences:

> *Many years later, as she was facing certain termination, Rachel Emmitt found herself remembering a distant time when her future looked more promising, and she was valued in the organization for her meticulous attention to detail.*

This sentence, however, would be tough to deliver on stage. Conversely, some spoken sentences work perfectly well when said aloud but would get a bad grade is sixth grade English class.

> *Did it matter? Yes! Did she care? Not a bit.*

Once you are pretty comfortable with your content, write a single word or phrase out in the margin like this:

bathroom scale — "When decorating my new home I bought a lot of new things including a bathroom scale. Now I had never owned a bathroom scale. I was always a skinny kid. Skinny kids don't own a bathroom scale. Why? Well, what's the use, really?

So now when you practice, you can look down and see this is where you tell the bathroom scale story. I usually write the note in bright red and in large enough letters that I can quickly read it from a distance.

> bathroom scale
> water bottle
> my father
> two years
> Nashville
> theater
> first job

With enough practice, you will be comfortable with this format, and you're mostly just relying on the single word or phrase in the margin. Now is the time to:

Transfer those words to an index card.
Depending on how long your talk is, you might have front and back of one index card, or you may have multiple cards. You can color code your cards for the beginning, middle, and end, or you can note on the corner the number.

Once you get to this point, the magic begins to happen. You are no longer reading; you are no longer memorizing. You are merely talking and occasionally referring back to your note cards. Now you can forget delivering your presentation flawlessly, word for word. Now you can talk because you *know* what you are going to say. Tell your first story and then your second story. Make your points. Transition through a couple of statistics and drive on to your big emotional close. The note cards are there if you need them, but as you progress you'll refer to them less and less.

Should you take note cards to the speaker's platform, whatever your platform is? Sure, why not? No one, not even professional newscasters, works without notes. Slide them out of your pocket and place them on a nearby stool or lectern. As you pause to take a moment to look down at your list and see where you are. No one cares if you brought notes.

What happens if you forget what comes next? Don't panic. Take a sip of water, flip through your notes, find your place, and resume. Done! No one died. Chances are good you are the only one who even noticed. What happens if you finish and suddenly it occurs to you that you forgot an entire section? Don't sweat it. You are the only one who knows your content, and the audience will never know what was left out.

A final point which seems to work for me: as you get closer to the day of your presentation try to practice at the same time of day that you'll be presenting. My brain seems to work remarkably better at some parts of the day than others. So, if next week I'm scheduled to speak from 9:00 a.m. to 10:30 a.m., this week I am practicing between 9:00 a.m. and 10:30 a.m. each day.

Three approaches to help people remember your presentation

How often have you heard a performance and you could not remember anything that was said? Conversely, do you ever look back and realize a piece of content you heard months or even years ago have still stayed with you? A compelling presentation is excellent, but a memorable presentation is even better. Here are three ways to ensure the audience remembers your content later.

Use acronyms

I was seventeen when I heard Zig Ziglar say, "Sometimes FEAR stands for 'False Evidence Appearing Real.'" Almost forty years later I still remember this because of the acronym. In music class, you likely heard, "Every Good Boy Does Fine" as an easy way to remember E, G, B, D, and F, the notes on the lines of a treble clef. You may have heard the acronym HOMES as an easy way to remember the Great Lakes: Huron, Ontario, Michigan, Erie, and Superior.

Acronyms are remarkable ways to jog your audience's memory. That's because acronyms, even bad ones, stick in your memory for years. How do you use them in your presentation? Look at your content and see if you can reorganize it into an acronym. Use an online synonym finder to discover alternate words that might fit your acronym. Let's say we want to teach supervisors to listen first, then reply. Can we make that fit into the acronym LEAD?

- **L**isten
- **E**mpathize
- Take **A**ction

Three letters were pretty easy, but "D?" What does that stand for? That's a bit of a struggle. After some research you might find, "Demonstrate." Does that work? You might suggest supervisors "LEAD" their teams, which means to "Listen" to them carefully, and "Empathize" with their struggles. Then "Take Action" when and where you can, and finally "Demonstrate" listening behaviors for your team. Will this acronym help them to remember? You bet. Try it now. Put this book down and do something else. In a few minutes ask yourself what the four behaviors we want supervisors to do are, and I'll bet you will remember all four.

Use an action

Your audience will be looking at facial expression, posture, body language, the tone of voice, and any physical movements to understand better what you are communicating. Consequently, an action- something you physically do while speaking- can be much easier to remember that the spoken word. Ask your audience to join you in an action:

> *Say, "Everybody clap." (Start clapping at a steady pace until your audience joins in. Each clap takes about one second.) "This year 480,000 Americans will die from smoking. If each time we clap represents one death, and another death and another, we'd have to clap for five days straight, twenty-four hours a day, to represent all smoking-related deaths this year."*

One of the presentations I like to share surrounds a concept in Quint Studer's bestselling book, *Results that Last*. Much of the book could be described as *what gets measured, gets moved*. I use the analogy of me stepping onto a bathroom scale after many years of not owning one. It goes something like this:

> *When decorating my new home, I bought a lot of new things including a bathroom*

scale. Now I had never owned a bathroom scale. I was always a skinny kid. Skinny kids do not own a bathroom scale. Why? Well, what's the use?

Then at the age of forty-five, I found myself shopping in house wares for a bathroom scale. I took one off the shelf, placed it on the floor and... *(I mime putting a bathroom scale on the floor and stepping onto it)* That number, *(pointing at the scale in disgust)* was not the number I was expecting. That scale was broken. I took another scale down to try out and it, too, was broken, as was the third and the fourth and the fifth. Each broken in the same way!

(I step away from where the scale is supposed to be on the floor and say to my audience:) By now, you are all probably thinking what I'm thinking. Right? How does a store like this stay in business? *(Audience laughs)*

Seriously... have you ever received a message you did not like, and blamed someone or something else for it? Were all the bathroom scales broken... alternatively;

was it possible, just a bit, that I was overweight?

That's much like the way we react when we get our patient satisfaction scores. What do we say? Oh! That measuring tool is broken. We step up (I mime stepping onto the scale) and blame the tool (pointing to the scale) instead of owning our results." (Hand to my chest, indicating myself)

My net result is my audience remembers me stepping onto, and then blaming the scale, so the next time they get a measurement or score they do not like, they will remember what I did in my presentation.

Keep your data current
Ask yourself regularly if you have the most current data. We just coached a team in Virginia whom all used ten-year-old data. When coached they located more current information and it significantly enhanced their talks. In fact, there is quite a bit of power in whipping out a statistic and saying, "As of this morning, 106,004 people have signed up."

Precise numbers beat vague numbers. Your audience won't be able to follow a long string of data, but when a statistic matters, *be accurate.*

> *Of the entire population of Americans with diabetes, 4.2 million, or 28.5%, will develop diabetic retinopathy.*

Many of us have trouble envisioning large complex numbers. A great follow up phrase is, "...which means..."

> *Of the entire population of Americans with diabetes, 4.2 million, or 28.5%, will develop diabetic retinopathy, which means, 4.2 million people are at risk of blindness, or about the same number of people as the population of Louisiana.*

Stay away from PowerPoint if possible
You've developed your big idea. You've researched statistics and information to back your premise. You're ready to sit down at PowerPoint, right? No, please do not. The more you can avoid PowerPoint the more your presentation will feel fresh. As soon as you boot it up you'll be seduced by the same old stale clichés that plague most presentations: bullet points, lofty-sounding quotes, blocks of text, and God

forbid, clip art. Don't go there if at all possible, but if you must, I have more to teach you in Chapter 14.

You are not the first
One mantra I always say to myself when trying to understand something is, "You are not the first." Whatever you are struggling with, there are hundreds and even thousands of others who have been there before. A quick look on Amazon and you find a dozen or more books on one subject. I am a huge fan of getting them all and synthesizing the best ideas quickly. Read with a highlighter and have sticky notes handy.

A feeling of hopelessness is common
At some point during my preparation, I am always overcome with the thought that none of this is any good, my presentation will be worthless, and I should not be allowed to speak. This feeling of hopelessness is normal, and you should always expect it.

Step away for a while
I like to go running; it clears my head. Along a stretch of highway running parallel to the beach, on a blistering August afternoon, as the sweat pours down my cheeks, I'm not thinking about my presentation-- I'm trying not to die from the heat.

I might go to a movie or shop at the farmer's market. Anything relatively mindless that will get me mentally away from my presentation for a period will work so I won't be *thinking* about it constantly. During those times of distractions, we are *thinking* about our presentation, but subconsciously. In the back of our mind, we are toying with the structure, the more important concepts, the stories, and sentences. Your subconscious mind is more likely to find random connections and odd choices than your conscious mind. This is what psychologists call the "Gestation Period."

Return with a fresh set of eyes
Now suddenly all of the missing pieces will be immediately clear. The weird structural questions will right themselves, your gaps will be showing, and you'll know what needs to happen next.

Do a 'you' or 'we' audit on your script
Write your script out entirely on a word processing program. Then do a 'you' or 'we' audit. That is, search your document for the words 'you' or 'we.' Your audience loves the words 'you' and 'we.' The more times you use those words, the more they feel included in the content. You *cannot* overuse the words 'you' and 'we.' Go back to any

section that isn't completely soaked in those terms and try to wedge a few more in. A more captive audience will reward you.

Be ready to remove some of the good stuff
We all fall in love with our *content*. We come across a quote, or a joke, or an inspirational piece and jam it into our presentation. Alone it may be excellent, beautiful, even stunning, but in the context of the entire section, it just may not fit.

It can be tough to *get rid of the good stuff.* Nonetheless, removing it is necessary unless it advances the entire presentation. Don't fall so in love with one piece that you damage the overall presentation by keeping it in.

The power of opposites
- "What began in doubt *ten years ago* ends in certainty *today.*"
- "Let's take this out of the *shadow* and celebrate it in the *sunshine.*"
- "When we consider what we did in the *past*, it is easy to have hope for our *future.*"

Contrasting a word or phrase with its opposite gives the sentence power.

The power of rhyme

- "We are more focused on our *goals* than we are in our *roles.*"
- "*Leaders* are *readers.*"
- "We ignored the *nurse* until our symptoms get *worse.*"

A rhymed word or phrase can take an ordinary sentence and make it extraordinary.

Alliteration creates more powerful sentences
- "The *poorer* the *patient*, the more *nurses* are *needed.*"
- "Whether we are in *Kalamazoo* or *Kansas*, we *seek* to *soothe* the *sickest.*"
- "It's not the *patients* who are the *problem.*"

Repeating the first sound is a traditional verbal technique that can add power to your phrases.

Metaphors make understanding quicker
- "It's like suddenly someone *turned on a spotlight*, and everyone could see all of our flaws."
- "This initiative has *remained in the starting gate* long after everyone else has *rounded the track.*"
- "The time to *learn to sail* is when the seas are calm."

Metaphors can make complex subjects easier to understand. We "fight" the good fight against "rogue cells" with a "silver bullet," hoping to "win the war" against the "enemy" disease.

Set them up before you say it
You can underline your key phrases by setting them up first. Instead of launching right into a line that you'll want your audience to remember, set it up with a line. "In my grandfather's office, centered on the wall over his big metal desk was this quote in a frame, 'It takes as much time to plan as it does to wish' by Eleanor Roosevelt.'" The setup is a way to call out the message to help them realize it is essential.

Keep track of them, they, and those
Sometimes your audience struggles to keep up with several people or thoughts you are covering unless you keep specific track of each.

For example, you refer to *administration, nurses, and housekeeping* while making your point. Then if you say *they* did something, your audience isn't sure which *they* you are talking about unless you clarify your statement.

Avoiding bookmarks in your presentation
When I read a good passage in a book, I turn over the page, highlight a line, or put a bookmark in that section. It allows me to move forward and back in the book comfortably. This technique does not work in a spoken presentation, however, but I hear many people try. They bring something

up and then declare, "I'm not going to cover that now, but this afternoon we'll get into it." Alternatively, "This tie into what I talked about at the beginning of my speech. Do you remember when I spoke about...?" Unlike a book, we cannot flip back to something earlier or turn over a page to remember it later. We cannot connect a piece of this morning's presentation with a part from the afternoon.

Humor in your presentation
Sandra was preparing for the one big presentation that would put her and her new division on the map. Getting attention often happens when your organization and career grow, and you suddenly find yourself on everyone's radar with invitations to present. Success in that single presentation can make the difference between a small division remaining small, or it can propel you to the next level.

Sandra called me saying a friend told her every good presentation is full of jokes. "Should I use humor in my presentation?" she asked. My answer was, "Humor, yes, but jokes, no."

Humor arises naturally out of your content and gives your audience a chance to see something in a humorous light. It's the part of your presentation said in a comedic way:

> My goal this week is to lose weight, so I'm trying a whole food diet - last night I ate a whole pizza.

Humor can lighten a serious presentation
Steve joined my class straight out of med school. He was a severe and sincere young man. The first presentation focused on his grandfather, a Marine, and a gift he gave Steve on his deathbed. Steve continued his story with some brief information about his father's death the previous year. Afterward, in a feedback session, I suggested he needed to lighten up his subject a bit. The following day in class Steve gave the same presentation, except this time he started with a joke:

> "What do you call cheese that does not belong to you?... nacho cheese!"

Steve then continued with his dead relatives' story. What I *should* have cautioned him about is that *one* dead relative is enough for an eight-minute presentation, and it would be better if he had left his father's death out. Humor should arise naturally from your content and never be pasted on as an afterthought.

The one person you can always make fun of is yourself

Self-deprecating humor is still the safest route and often helps your audience feel better about themselves. They may not feel confident in a particular skill, but at least they are better than you once were. Making fun of your younger, less confident self endears you to your audience.

> *"I struggled with procrastination, and for years I put off asking for help.*
>
> *While out for a run, I was back after two minutes because I forgot something- I forgot that I'm so out of shape I cannot run more than two minutes."*

Jokes can be quicksand

A joke is a story composed of a setup and a punch line that feels pasted on. A joke stops your presentation, instead of taking your audience into a different place with that predictable format of setup followed by the punch line.

> Joke: Two blondes decided to split a can of Diet Coke. One blonde opened the can and poured half the contents into her glass and

> half into her friend's glass. Before tossing the can, she stopped to read the nutritional information on the side. "Only one calorie per can," she read out loud. "Hm," murmured the other blonde. "I wonder which glass has the calorie?"

Most jokes make fun of someone, like the "blondes" in the example above. If you do this, your chances of offending someone are very real. My friend Jeremy spoke to a group of dental assistants in Nashville. Jeremy had been through a rough divorce, and he peppered his presentation with ex-wife jokes. The first few jokes brought out a few groans from his audience, but towards the end, I thought a few of the women in the audience were ready to punch him. Jeremy has never been back to Nashville.

Any joke or comment that is even remotely sexist, racist, homophobic or dirty has no place in your presentation. None whatsoever.

Common phrases like "red-headed stepchild" can offend as well. If you think someone might be offended, take it out. Have someone listen as you practice and specifically ask them to tell you if anything sounds offensive.

Sometimes potentially offending words or phrases can be well hidden from you because they are so much a part of the vernacular. I remember a training session I was facilitating when one of the presenters talked about the problems "managing up" her boss. "The reason we do not do it," she suggested, "is because it feels like brown-nosing." It had never occurred to her what brown-nosing meant. When others in the class pointed it out to her, she was mortified and changed it right away.

A friend told us a story of a nurse leader who was presenting to upper management of an extensive hospital system. This nurse leader had a photo of her daughter in her slide presentation. She was rightly proud of her daughter, who had achieved significant success as a world-class gymnast, a finalist for the Olympic team, and a cheerleader for a pro sports team. Who wouldn't be proud of that? However, when the slide popped up, what the audience saw was a beautiful, voluptuous blonde in a skimpy mini skirt and halter-top.

The system's CEO abruptly walked out, and a chill fell across the meeting. To the nurse leader, it was a picture of her amazing daughter. To the CEO it was a racy picture of a blonde bombshell. The lesson here is to check your work. Ask others to view your presentation ahead of time. Permit them to tell you when something seems off. Think about the most sensitive person who might see your presentation and what might offend them.

Any departure from your presentation can be disastrous for your intent. Your presentation is a journey, taking people from where they are to where you want them to be. Using inappropriate or offensive words or media can be the death knell.

A checklist

Is your message aligned? Does your message match with what others in the organization are saying? Does it successfully match the information expressed in other departments and at different levels? Communication is most potent when it cascades from leader to leader and when all divisions hear a similar message at the same time.

Do you remember the game of "telephone?" In this game, one person would whisper into the ear of another, who would then whisper to the next and the next and the next. The final message the final person in the chain hears would usually be dramatically different from the original message. It's funny as a childhood game but a disaster in a large organization.

It's usually a good idea to check with other leaders and see how they are positioning the information with their teams. Aligned messages are powerful in moving an organization forward. It is for this reason we often train in groups. If two leaders from the same group express dramatically different messages, they bog an organization down. When they teach together, they have a better chance of being aligned.

Are you starting close to the action? I cannot stress this strongly enough. Most talks begin so weakly that by the time they get to the substance, the audience is no longer paying attention. You have at most thirty seconds to answer their question, "What's in this for me?" Answer that forcefully in the opening paragraph.

Example: a weak opening

> *"I want to thank you all for being here. Last month when Dave and I were in Nashville, we talked about allowing me to address your team...."*

Do you see? There is nothing there to benefit the audience.

Example: a much stronger opening
> *"Between 700,000 and 1 million patients have a fall during their hospital stays in U.S. hospitals. It's a trauma for the patients and their families, and it's a trauma for you, the care team. Today we're exploring some tactics to reduce that number."*

Immediately the speaker begins by addressing a concern of everyone in the room along with a promise of how to improve.

Do I illustrate my main points with stories? People will forget your bullet points minutes after you leave but a clear story will stay with them forever. In the above example about hospital falls we can make the statistic real by telling about a nurse who finds a patient on the floor. One story about one person can be more powerful than a number on a PowerPoint slide.

Have I made sure my PowerPoint is *not* the star of the show? PowerPoint can help to illustrate your points, but it can also be a distraction, mainly when you play to the slides rather than to the audience.

We see this all of the time. With the first few slides the presenter is still addressing the audience, but over time the gravitational pull of the slide deck replaces eye contact between presenter and audience. Instead of connecting with the audience, even the presenter is watching "the show." The slides become the star, the presenter becomes secondary, and the audience is forgotten.

Visuals support your story; they are not your story. If you let the PowerPoint be the driver, you will lose your audience every time.

Have I provided some proof? Healthcare leaders are steeped in science and science is based on evidence. You may be charming, likable, and smart, but without some proof of your contentions people rightly may resist your conclusions. In most cases, you do not need page after page of carefully collated data, but you need something...at least a bar graph with a citation.

Do I ask for and receive feedback from the audience as I go along?
>"Does this make sense?"
>"Are you with me on this?"
>"This has probably happened to you, right?"
>"How would you have handled that?"

This sort of call-and-response speaking style keeps the audience engaged. Especially when you give the audience time to think about their answer and respond, even if it's just a head nod.

Do I alert them to key takeaways? Out of everything you say you likely have a few key takeaways you want the audience to remember later. Call those items out with a direct appeal. "Now, here is the most important point you should remember. If you get one thing from this talk, this is it."

Have I removed industry jargon and unnecessary acronyms? We love our acronyms, do not we? Most hospital units are filled with CCU's and OPD's. However, this endless acronym cascade can be hard for everyone to follow. If there is a possibility that even a single audience member does not know a term or acronym, leave it out. Yes, it does take a few seconds more to say "Cardiac Care Unit" or "Outpatient Department" rather than the acronym, but you have a better chance of everyone following your presentation without industry jargon and acronyms.

Do I talk regarding 'we' and 'us' instead of 'you'? "You'll need to... also, when rounding make sure you..." can sound preachy. If instead, you say, "When we are rounding we automatically do an environmental assessment, right?" then it sounds less bossy and more inclusive.

The value of an introduction
Before you even begin your presentation, you want your audience to know that you have something important to say and that your knowledge and prior experiences will lend credence to your message. You do not want to begin your speech by telling them these things yourself. An introducer can say things about you, describing your background, your interests, and your accomplishments, which you cannot say without seeming immodest.

Always ask to be introduced
Why? Your introduction will set you up for success. Years ago, an organization I worked with asked me to speak at a training event. I asked the event organizer to introduce me, and she laughed, "But, Daniel, these people already know who you are." That was not the point. Even though they knew me, at that moment I wanted to be seen in the best possible light, not just the guy in the break room talking about his weekend. So, I was introduced, and after my presentation I had co-

workers come to me and say, "We had no idea the things you've done before joining the company."

Write your introduction
Take the time to write out your introduction. If the introducer does it, you may not be described from the most advantageous perspective for you. Write it explicitly for *that event* and *that crowd*. There is no need to put all of your accomplishments in this intro, just those relevant to that day's mission. If you're speaking about leadership, talk about your previous leadership experience. If your subject is growing tomatoes, use information about growing up on a farm.

Send the introduction ahead of time, but also bring it with you
Create one-page (at the most) introduction in at least a fourteen-point font, so it is easy to read with or without glasses. Send it to your host ahead of time and then bring a copy with you. Your host may forget or lose the original, so your printed copy saves the day.

Always stand up when speaking
Scientists tell us most of our communication is nonverbal, so stand up! Actor Denzel Washington considered declining an offer to star in the movie *The Bone Collector* because he wasn't sure he

could command the audience's attention from a seated position, which the role required. Now I do not know about you, but if Denzel Washington struggles to command attention seated, what chance do the rest of us have? If your audience cannot see you, they are only getting at most thirteen percent of what you are saying. If they cannot see you *and* they're having trouble hearing you, too, you have dramatically reduced your effectiveness. Even if the fifteen people who speak before you do not stand up or the fifteen people who speak after you do not stand up, *you need to stand up* while you speak - every time, always.

Move to the center of the room

No matter what, move from where you are to the center of the room so that everyone can see you. This is the strongest part of the room. It suggests authority and confidence.

I recently spoke to a group of nonprofit directors in Atlanta. They received all of the information I shared with them well, and they were soon ready to role-play some of the major points we had talked about. However, their natural shyness made it difficult for them to take a position on a stage that looked so dominant. It was just way too intimidating. Finally, a young woman named DeeDee agreed to try it. She strode from the very back row to the front of the room. She looked out at the audience with her hands casually placed at about her beltline. She smiled a bit and made eye contact with a number of the people in the room. Then slowly she began to speak. "There are three things...," she said in a broad, clear voice, and the audience applauded. DeeDee suddenly looked like she owned the place. This is the look of authority you need to have.

Hands in front

During my time in television, I've put more than ten thousand people on camera. What was their number one question for me? "What do I do with my hands?" At one time my answers would have been vague. "Try this," I would advise, "or maybe this would work." Over time, however, I've become much more prescriptive; I only want you to do one thing. Put your hands together right in front of your waistline. Hold your hands loosely and make eye contact. Keep your hands at your waist area when you rest between gestures like this:

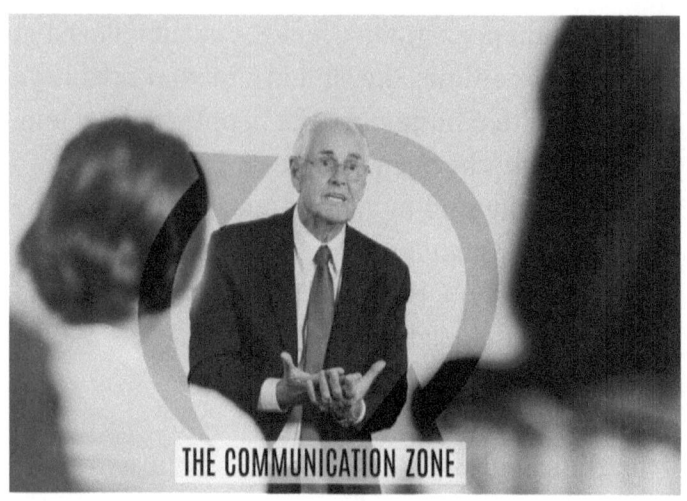
THE COMMUNICATION ZONE

Being likable and trustworthy
First stride to the front of the room making eye contact with a few key people. Pause and smile. More and more I'm convinced that a big smile is a superpower. Eye contact signals you can trust me. Smiling signals that you like them. Science has shown that when people look at each other, they subconsciously sync their mood with the other person. If I am smiling when you meet me, you are more likely to smile as well.

Not all smiles are about showing teeth; some we hear in your voice. Next time you are around someone who is genuinely happy listen to his or her tone. Look for videos on YouTube of people who are newly engaged or who have won money, or kids who've just been told they are going to

Disneyland. Hear that tone and try to replicate it in your voice.

Using gestures
A research study tried to understand why some TED Talk videos got millions of views and others received very few views. They discovered that the most popular TED Talks videos were the ones where the speaker gestured all the time. In fact, some of the most watched speakers gestured more than three hundred and fifty times in eighteen minutes, while the least watched speakers gestured less than one hundred times in the same amount of time.

Often my clients will comment on how much they are gesturing and think their hands are somehow distracting. Just the opposite is true. If most of your communication is nonverbal then gestures are not *distracting* from your message, gestures are *communicating* your message. Keep your hands in your Communication Zone so your gestures will be small and direct attention back to your face instead of around the room.

Use specific gestures
Best use of gestures to keep your audience engaged:

Point with a hand, not a finger
Many consider pointing your finger at someone to be a rude gesture. Instead, indicate with a flat hand, not your finger, to your audience. They understand you're referring to them. Use of a flat hand is like reaching out with a handshake.

You, me, and we
Refer to an audience member with a flat hand, and then to yourself, then bring your hands back together again.

Illustrate a number
Whenever possible gesture your number when you say it. Four? (Hold up four fingers) Three parts of a problem? (Hold up three fingers) Once again, your nonverbal help the audience to follow what you are saying.

Physically communicate your emotions
Anytime you touch yourself in the heart region of your torso, it communicates your emotional connection to the subject. Try it now. Say, "this is important to me" without a hand gesture. Now say the same thing while touching your heart. That is far more powerful, isn't it?

Bring things together
You can establish a specific item or group in your right hand, and another in your left hand. Bring your hands together to demonstrate agreement.

> "So, the housekeeping staff finally got what they wanted" (hold up your left hand) "and then the care team got what they wanted" (hold up your right hand) "and suddenly these two groups came together" (move your hands together to illustrate).

Increase and decrease
When you say something goes up, accompany that statement with a hand gesture that moves up as well. As something goes down, bring your hand down at the same time.
If something gets larger, bring your hands out from the center. If you say something is tiny, make a gesture by holding your thumb and forefinger close together and squint your eyes through your fingers.

Culturally specific gestures

In most of America, we understand a few basic gestures such as thumbs up, okay, door knocking, and the blown kiss. Be careful, however, because other cultures do not always have the same meaning for these gestures. For instance, the 'thumbs up' gesture in the Middle East can be seen as offensive. Therefore, it is crucial to understand the makeup of your audience. If you find yourself speaking to a group of foreigners or even Americans who are the first generation, you may need to adapt your gestures not to cause any offense.

Monotone is the death of engagement

If we all sat around and watched a bunch of bad presentations, the most common criticism would be *monotone*. Nothing kills engagement more rapidly than speaking in a monotone of voice. Monotone robs your audience of your content. Even the most well-meaning audience member will find their attention drifting when listening to a speaker who says every sentence and every word with the same flat affect. What can we do to prevent such a horrid fate? Plenty! Here are some tools you can use right away to get and keep the audience's attention.

Vary your tone

Tone refers to the audible pitch of your voice. It's not important what your natural pitch is, but that you *vary your pitch*. To illustrate let's imagine picking up your child at the car line at school. You ask, "What did you do today?" "Nothing." "What did you learn?" "I don't know." Can you hear that tone in your head right now? That's a flat tone. Then one day you pick up your child and

Closed body language hides the torso from others by crossing your arms and legs to protect your most vulnerable core. Your head is down protecting your neck, your hands are hidden, and you may position your body toward an open door, and away from the person, you are talking to. Nonverbally you are saying, "I do not trust you, you're not my friend."

Confident body language means making yourself larger, keeping your chin up, standing straight and tall, gesturing with your palms up and your hands always visible, and making eye contact. Nonverbally you are saying, "I got this."

Nervous body language diminishes you, making yourself smaller. You cross your arms in a protective gesture across your body, put your chin down, fail to make or sustain eye contact. You may engage in self-comfort gestures like playing with your hair or rubbing your hands against each other.

Humans naturally sync up with one another, initially by reading each other's body language. If you demonstrate nervousness to your audience, they will feel it, too, and become anxious as well. If you show confidence in your body language, your audience will sync up with you and will also feel confident. Open, confident people are easier to like. Why? When we are with them, we tend to feel more open and confident ourselves. We like ourselves better when we are open and confident.

However, what if you do not feel confident? You can try Amy Cuddy's Power Poses. Amy Cuddy is a Harvard researcher and social psychologist who gave a Ted Talk that has gone on to be viewed more than thirty-nine million times. In her talk, she says you can change your confidence level by merely changing your body language. Doing what she calls "power poses" for as little as two minutes changes your body chemistry, reducing your cortisol (stress hormone) and increasing your testosterone (confidence hormone). We've done power poses in many of our classes and participants are convinced it changes how everyone feels.

Be aware of your body language throughout

As a part of my wife's business, she visits with restaurant owners and managers. The best time to chat with them is usually just before they open or during the quieter parts of the afternoons. That said, when Donna drives up she is often the only car in the parking lot, and she is aware the owners and managers are watching her from the time she enters the lot. How she looks and handles herself matters even when she is still out in the parking lot.

I'm working with a young clinic director, Tyler, who looks perfect when he is in front of a group. He leans forward, has excellent gestures and makes good eye contact. However, the moment Tyler steps to the back of the room he slouches and shoves his hands into his pockets. Your body language matters even when you are not in front of a group. Your hands should never be in your pockets. Ever.

We are currently coaching a small team of leaders who will present as a group in a few months. When they are standing, body language is perfect. When they are sitting, however, they tend to look bored or even angry. Remember, you are 'on stage' from the moment you arrive in the parking lot until you have driven away at the end. What you do in the coffee line outside the room may matter more than when you're in front of the room.

One final cautionary tale on this subject. Years ago, our company was trying to hire a new executive, and we thought we'd found the best fit. As he came in for a second interview, he was rude to the person at the front desk. The executive team conducting the interviews met in a room with a window overlooking the lobby. We watched him make angry gestures, throw his coat down, and point at the receptionist. He did not get the job. The best bet is to remember you are on stage the entire time, not just after you've stepped on stage.

Write out your presentation

Write out your complete presentation, then go back and annotate times when you will speak slowly and other times when you will speak fast. This will enable you to grasp and keep your audience's attention. Note when to pause, whisper or get loud, like this:

>   *very slowly*
> There is only one thing we need to
>   *pause*
> consider today. One thing. In boardrooms
>   *said with increasing intensity and speed*
> like this we like to make ourselves feel
>   *said with increasing intensity and speed*
> important by solving big important problems.
> *pause*   *hit every word and pause between*
> ✓But today it is simple. Incredibly simple.
>   *almost in a whisper*
> Today we have to solve physician engagement

Use the entire stage

My experience shows there are two types of presenters: those who lock in on one place on the stage and never move, and those that continuously pace like the Bengal Tiger in the San Diego Zoo. Neither technique works to engage your audience.

Cheryl is a young leader of a mid-sized medical group, and her immediate supervisor thought she might benefit from having some coaching. One-on-one she was bright and engaging, but on stage, she froze. We have a videotape of Cheryl presenting at a conference where she not only froze, but she positioned herself at the furthest back part of the stage next to the monitor in almost total darkness, and she never moved once during her presentation. Needless to say, she did not receive an excellent evaluation from that breakout.

The opposite is an early tape of me presenting. I am embarrassed to say I nervously paced from one end of the stage to the other without cessation for the entire hour. My Fitbit for that hour showed I walked almost six thousand steps!

Much like the previous advice about varying your tone, volume and pace, moving about on stage can add interest to your presentation, but you should walk with purpose and not randomly as I did.

Imagine going to a stage play and seeing the actors stand on stage in one location and never moving. How boring would that be? Theater directors know that to maintain the audience's interest they need to move the actors within the available space. They also understand different positions on stage mean different things. So, let's talk about how this applies to our work as presenters.

Center stage right in front is the power position. We start there because it gives us the most authority. Nonverbally we establish our authority by:

- Taking up space,
- Standing in silence
- Presenting ourselves in symmetry
- Speaking and moving slowly
- Maintaining our stillness

Early in our presentations we move to the center of the space, stand symmetrically, pause before speaking and move and speak slowly. This is what leadership looks like. Our goal right out of the gate is to dominate the stage and demand the attention.

In almost every case your best move is to stride comfortably to center stage, stand still and make eye contact with key audience members, and pause for at least four seconds before you begin.

Signal chapter headings

In a book like this one, there are visual cues when we change subjects. When the chapter changes, there is a space followed by a headline before beginning the new content. We do the same thing on stage by taking a 'chapter' break between subjects.

In our case, we might talk about the big picture problem from our power position center stage. When we want to transition to a more emotional story of how this affects a real person, we move downstage, closer to the audience. Couple that move with more open and approachable body language and your audience will understand we're moving to a new part of our presentation.

So, we might stage our talk like this:
- Open, center stage, the big picture about the problem and why you should care, transition to:
- Emotional story, how this problem affects one person, we move down nearer to the audience and use a more intimate tone, transition to:
- Stage left, a discussion about early failed attempts to solve the problem, transition to:
- Stage right, other additional steps taken to alleviate the problem, transition to:
- Center stage again discussing solutions that work, transition to:
- Downstage again near the audience when we talk about a connect to purpose story of one person or one family as the problem is solved and how their lives are improved because of that.

This use of the entire stage captures and keeps the audience's attention plus it signals when you change subjects. We use the more emotional intimate space down near the audience to speak of emotional stories, and we use the center stage to establish our authority.

One caution, however. You should move deliberately and with purpose. This isn't a 'wander around and land' process; it is a deliberate process with planned impact.

Another note to be aware of: You should not deliver important information *while you are walking*. It's okay to talk as you shift position, but when you hit your main points, you should be still to give them the power they deserve. It goes like this, "What made this leader powerful?" (Move to the next position). "Optimism. Belligerent, outrageous, unmitigated optimism."

Never use the lectern

Imagine this: a non-profit director is preparing for the most significant presentation of his life, and he is terrified, like white-knuckled, shortness-of-breath terrified. Luckily for him, he has assembled a team to prepare him for the event. He has a writer, an artist creating the

PowerPoint, a colleague who manages the event, and an on-site event manager and the team at a large ballroom in Miami. He also brought me on to coach him on speaking skills. We had two months to get him ready.

We drilled him on every step, over and over and over. I called the event organizer on site, and I made sure of one thing.... there can be NO LECTERN in the room. I think I asked for that four times.

We arrive and what is right in the middle of the stage? A massive wooden lectern. The director loves it and insists we keep it. Okay... now imagine the day of this big presentation. The director strides onstage with a pile of notes and stands at the lectern. He lowers his head and reads for four and a half hours. For four and a half hours the only thing we see is the top of his head and his knuckles, as he holds onto the lectern for dear life. It was a disaster.

I always ask for the lectern to be removed when I speak. Our audience needs to see our full body. They need to see our gestures. We need to move around as we talk. As soon as you are anchored to a lectern, none of this is possible.

Note about microphones

You will likely encounter one of four microphone situations:
- No microphone at all
- A microphone attached to the lectern
- A handheld microphone
- A lavalier microphone

Ask the event organizer this question ahead of time. Given a choice, I always ask for a lavalier microphone. A lavalier microphone or lav mic is a tiny, inconspicuous microphone that attaches to your tie or shirt up near your collar. You've likely seen newscasters on TV wearing these. For a speaker this is ideal because you do not have to hold it and you can use your hands to gesture, open water bottles, flip through note cards.

The one downside of a lavalier microphone is that the battery pack has to attach to your belt or fit in a pocket. Some women's clothing lacks both a pocket and a belt...but the battery pack has to go *somewhere*. I've seen women have to go to the restroom and get a colleague to attach the battery pack to their bra strap. This not ideal for many reasons. Also, women should be aware that their necklaces might brush against the microphone. Dangly necklaces, scarves, and long hair can brush against the microphone, making a distracting sound. When you arrange to speak somewhere, make a note in your day planner to wear an outfit with a belt or pockets and keep jewelry around your neck to a minimum.

The handheld microphone, the type that many comedians use, is an excellent second choice. A significant advantage is you can move it up close to your mouth when talking or put it down to your side when you're having a one-on-one conversation. There are two downsides, however. It can get heavy if you speak for a long time. I've held a handheld for an hour, and my shoulder began to feel it over time. The other downside is you cannot use that hand for anything else. If you have a bottle of water, reading glasses, a note card and a prop on stage, it can be a lot to juggle with one hand.

In small groups, you may opt for no microphone at all. I find I can communicate well in a room of about fifty people without a microphone, but my voice is rather loud. Depending on how powerful your voice is, your mileage may vary. In a larger group, if you are straining to be heard, your voice will wear out more quickly. No microphone, in that case, can work against you.

Finally, let's talk about the dreaded lectern. I try to work with the event organizer to get a lavalier microphone if at all possible. Sometimes they will tell you that the mic on the lectern is the only choice, but when you persist, they discover their AV people have a lavalier or handheld microphone as well. It does not hurt to ask. However, sometimes a lectern is your only choice. If the event is small enough you might still be able to speak loudly enough not to need the microphone.

The only way I've seen to overcome the disadvantages of the lectern partially is to stand slightly apart from it. Leaning on a podium is just dreadful. Stand back so that you can still gesture and move around a bit but staying just close enough to the microphone to be heard. Ask the audience if they can listen to you and the AV person if they can turn the lectern microphone up a bit.

Your microphone is always on

We always have to assume that our microphone is on. That means from the moment you are given a microphone you must be very careful what you say. We had a presenter in Louisville step off the stage and quickly exit into the hallway; not realizing her microphone was still on. She said loud enough for the entire ballroom to hear, "God, that was awful!" It takes discipline to learn to respect the microphone, but we have to do it. Never assume you are "off." Always assume anything you say can be heard in the room. Many an ex-politician has learned this lesson the hard way.

Step Six

Show Some Statistics

We watched a dynamite presentation from our colleagues in Australia, but something seemed amiss. Because it had been recorded we watched it over and over a few times. That's when the problem occurred to us. "Maggie is your presentation based on evidence or is it just your opinion?" Maggie assured us her presentation was based on reliable scientific data but, because she didn't share any of that data, we were left wondering.

Currently, as part of our work with nonprofits, we are teaching a large group of speakers who are focused on the problem of human trafficking. Every training session I ask over and over again, how big of a problem is this? How often does it happen? How many victims are there? Is the problem getting better or worse? Without some statistical information, it's going to impossible for an audience to know how concerned they should be. If it's twenty people in the United States each year, we may not be that concerned. If it's 20,000, then we are right to be focused on solving the problem.

Whenever possible utilize at least one scientific looking graphic. Scientists at Cornell found a paragraph about medication was only 67% effective in convincing the reader. However, the same paragraph when accompanied by a 'scientific looking' graphic suddenly was 96.6% effective *even though the graphic contained no new information.* This effect is widely believed to be due to an audience's belief in the validity of scientific information.

Stephanie understands how vital a few carefully chosen PowerPoint slides can be. She is a coach who works with tough financial management clients in healthcare. Many times, her clients are not happy to see her, and in fact, quite often her audience can be openly hostile to her. However, Stephanie isn't shy about sharing her information. She'll state that half of all hospitals are losing money on patient care. Then she'll follow up with a slide from Health Affairs that shows 55% of all hospitals lose money on patient care and one-third of all US hospitals make less than $1000 on each discharged patient. Over and over when she speaks she'll say something, the audience thinks, "I don't believe that!" and then she follows up with a graphic to prove her point. After that's happened many times, the audience begins to believe Stephanie knows what she's talking about.

Make numbers easier to understand

Numbers can be hard to understand in a spoken form. There are four ways to help your audience follow:

Repeat the number.

If I hit a number in my presentation, I'll usually say it at least twice.

> "Twenty-three percent of all hospitals in Ohio are losing money or are operating on a margin of less than 2%. That's amazing, right? 23% of all hospitals."

Be repeating the number your audience has more than a single chance to catch it.

Round off the number.

Complex numbers can be challenging to get our mind around when only shared verbally. It helps to round off the number to make it easier to understand.

> "In American how many people are living with HIV/AIDS? As of today, 468,578. Almost half a million people."

Show it AND say it.

If you put the numbers up on a PowerPoint slide and say them out loud, the audience has a better chance of getting it. Indeed, if your presentation contains multiple numbers a PowerPoint slide deck can help your audience follow along.

Compare the number to one we can more easily relate to

> "About 1.5 million people are in hospice care in the US. To give you some idea of how large that population is...if we put all of the people receiving hospice care into one area it would be the fifth largest city in the US."

In the end, I'll leave you with this; the old saying goes,

One hundred thousand deaths are a statistic. One death...when it is your mother...is a tragedy.

No matter how significant the number is trying to personalize it with a single person's story.

Step Seven

Finish Strong

Because of the Recency Effect, your audience will be most likely to remember your close, and so that's where we put a lot of our time and effort.

In most cases we want the open and close of your speech to be memorized word-for-word. They are too important to 'wing it.'

Reflect back on the open

The open and close are 'bookends' for your speech, and quite often we want them to look and feel the same. If you opened with your grandfather's experience in hospice, you might want to close with a completion of that story. If you began your talk with this quote from Teddy Roosevelt:

> *"Nothing in the world is worth having or worth doing unless it means effort, pain, difficulty. I have never in my life envied a human being who has led an easy life. I have*

> envied a great many people who have led difficult lives and led them well."

Then you might come back at the end and reflect that message.

> "If we believe like Teddy Roosevelt did that nothing worth doing is without effort pain and difficulty, then we will be ready for the challenges we face. Also, perhaps someday we will say about our own lives...we led difficult lives, and we led them well."

Find your inspirational voice

The closing paragraphs are your chance to be inspirational. This is a chance to step back and look at the 30,000-foot view. This is a chance to go beyond the everyday dullness of so much of our talks, and to reach out and inspire the group.

> "I will remind you there will be doubters. There will be tough times. There will be mistakes, and there will be disappointments. However, if we do the right things, for the right reasons, at the right time, we will prevail. So, one day we will stand here and say, 'we did this. We did. We made this happen.' I am proud to be working with you all."

End with a call to action

In the end, what is it that you want the group to do? It's usually a good idea to say that out loud before you close. What action should they take? What are the next steps? Be concrete and specific.

> *"I know we've covered a lot...and no doubt you'll have questions. Take my number and Mark's number and please call us with questions. Moreover, when we're together again next month, we'll spend some time just going through all the questions and concerns we've heard."*

Question and Answer sessions can be a minefield

Not every presentation needs a question and answer period. I know a Chief Nursing Officer who prepared a marvelous presentation. She was funny, smart, and personable, but what worried her the most was how to handle the Q&A session. All too often a brilliant presentation is brought down by an off the subject, confrontational, or even hostile question. If a question is unanticipated by the speaker, that, too, can derail an otherwise effective presentation. Decide whether a Q&A session is appropriate to the topic or even necessary, as there may be other ways to follow up on the information conveyed by the speaker. In the case of the CNO, she contacted the event manager ahead of time and learned that the Q&A period was available only if desired and was, therefore, optional.

If your topic necessitates a question and answer session, bury it in your presentation. Do not close with it. Why? Too often you may get a question that is off-topic, bizarre or posed in such a way that a hostile environment ensues. Any of these situations may cause *that* to be remembered more than your closing.

So, you say, "Before I close I'd like to answer a few short questions. Now we only have a few minutes until we break so let's save the most complex questions until after lunch. Let me take a couple of questions now and then I'll come back and close our morning with a few final thoughts." This establishes that question and answers time will be short. Longer and more complex questions will be answered but later, and you've told them you would retake the floor at the end for some final thoughts.

At some point toward the end of your presentation announce you will be taking about five or six questions now, but then come back at the end to close. Your audience will remember your closing statement rather than an off-the-wall question.

To ensure your Q&A session goes well, give the audience warning that you are going to take questions. Some in the audience will encounter problems they want to ask even as you are addressing that topic; others need time to construct what they are going to ask. You might say, "In a few minutes I'll answer some questions so be thinking about what questions you may have."

When no one has any questions

Imagine a ballroom in a large city. The presenter on stage is speaking about her newly-released book. Perhaps one hundred and fifty people sit in the first few rows. The presenter is good. She talks about why she wrote the book, what the key takeaways are, who the intended audience is. She finishes with a heartwarming story that builds to an emotional close that manages to include the book's title. Beautiful. Then she makes a fatal error. After a bit of applause, she asks, "Are there any questions?" Unfortunately, awkward silence ensues, until she sheepishly says, "Okay, then I'll sign some books." That extended silence robs her presentation of all of its punch.

What could she have done differently? Of course, she could not have taken questions. However, she could have also planted a question or two in the audience. After all, many in the audience might be friends or colleagues. There is nothing wrong with asking a friend, "Hey, when we do the question and answer period, would you mind asking me about this..." and then planting a good question with that person.

Newscasters do this all the time. The reporter in the field will call in ahead with their story, and the anchor will ask, "What is a good question for me to ask you?" This makes for a great exchange during the show. The reporter concludes her report, the anchor fires back with an insightful question, and the reporter gives a perfectly prepared answer. It not only makes for an excellent way to end the story, but it also helps the audience because usually, the anchor is asking a question the audience at home would like to ask.

Because of the "Recency Effect," the way you close will be the most memorable part of the presentation. As your audience returns to their work environments, they will discuss your final words more than what you have said in the middle of your presentation. You want those last words to be meaningful as well as memorable. If you close with a Q&A period, the final words could be awkward, testy, or off-topic, and that could undermine the effectiveness of the entire talk.

The Tough Questions exercise

There are times when you know your audience may not just be skeptical; they may be openly hostile. Several times I have worked with elected officials and city leaders needing help in communicating policy decisions to the public, or with business teams who are facing layoffs and restructuring within their organizations. These can be tough times for clear communications.

If you know or suspect you are going to be facing difficult questions, you and your team should prepare ahead of time.

Step one is to make a list of probable tough questions. If your organization is merging or restructuring, most questions may arise out of fear of people losing their jobs. Politicians always have a handful of hot-button political issues that will be asked. The secret here is to realize that, although these questions may be challenging to answer, they are seldom unexpected. Use the preparation process with your team to craft thoughtful responses to your most anticipated questions.

Make sure you and other leaders in the organization are in alignment with your answers. Fear kicks the rumor and gossip into high gear. If one leader is saying one thing and another is saying something else, employees may not believe anything they are being told. Bring all the leaders into the same room and practice. Your internal alignment can be vital to reducing anxiety.

Step two is to use reflective listening skills to demonstrate that you are listening.

> *Questioner: "How do you know there won't be layoffs in my department after we merge?"*
> *Leader: "You are concerned about possible layoffs after the merger? Did I understand the question correctly?"*

Keep clarifying their question until they feel like you understood it accurately. This may take several steps with difficult and emotional issues like layoffs. Don't stop when you *think* you know their concerns. Quit only when they are *confident* you understand.

Quite often the reason people ask questions is that they want their leader to hear them and validate their concerns. The content of your answer may not be as valuable as demonstrating that you are listening, and you take their interests seriously. Follow up with a statement that validates their concerns. "I understand why you are worried. Times like this can be unsettling. You are right to bring this up."

Speak slower and with precision. Your audience may want to parse your words and to listen to not just what you say but the way you say it. Avoid anything that reeks of sleek smooth-talking and insincerity. If you get a question you do not know the answer to, now is not the time to make something up. Tell them you do not know.

Communicate more when tough questions arise. Spend more time on the tough questions than on questions when everyone is happy. Emotional moments require more communication and more frequent communication.

Bonus Chapter

PowerPoint Success

Former Vice President Al Gore took the world by storm with his presentation, *An Inconvenient Truth*, chronicling the effects of climate change around the world. The presentation became a documentary that won two Academy Awards, and Gore was awarded the Nobel Peace Prize in 2007. That's pretty snazzy for what amounts to, primarily, a PowerPoint presentation.

Business in America runs on PowerPoint. I worked with one company so addicted to the technology that I do not think they could talk about their weekend plans without a slide advancer and slide deck. "Here's the beach we will go to, (click) and the bar where we'll have margaritas."

The lure of PowerPoint

We try to talk leaders out of using slide presentation software because, more often than not, it gets in the way of communicating with the audience and establishing a real connection.

We see it all the time. A presenter begins with a real focus on message and audience. Click, the first slide. The speaker briefly looks toward the screen to explain the slide. Click, the second slide. Now it begins the slow turn away from the audience to address the content of the PowerPoint. Click, the third slide. Even more complex information appears on the slide, and the presenter entirely disconnects from the audience and locks in on the PowerPoint. Click, click, and click through to the end. Presenters who make this error almost never maintain eye contact with their audience. Instead, all of their attention is on the slides. The audience and the presenter co-read the slides line-by-line and word-by-word. PowerPoint seems almost to have a gravitational pull. The closer you get to it the more you are sucked into it until you can no longer pull away.

Make your audience the star

Your audience is the star, and your message is the critical mass. If the totality of that message ends up on a slide deck, nothing else matters, not the audience, not you, nothing but what's on the slides. When we advise, "Never make your PowerPoint the star," we mean that you should use the slide deck *only* to illustrate what is difficult to describe with the spoken word alone.

Recently I worked with a group who was furiously preparing for a critical presentation, and they were stuck. When I inquired what the hold up was, they said, "On this slide, we need a picture of the fire, and no one seems to have one." Some years ago, their clinic had burned along with a row of other buildings. It was a tragedy that almost sank their fledgling operation. They were stuck because they assumed a photo on a slide *must* illustrate an event of that magnitude. Of course, this was not the case. After all, we've all seen fires; we have no trouble imagining what a fire looks like. If you watch the evening news, you are more likely than not to see a couple of local fires presented. Was their fire different? In some small ways, but those differences can be easily communicated in the spoken dialogue. In fact, I would contend their final presentation was more powerful because of the *lack* of a photo of the fire.

In the end, this is how they handled their presentation. The speaker showed beautiful pictures of the clinic being built and the day it opened. These were large, professional-quality photos. The audience understood why they were proud of their work. Suddenly, instead of advancing to the next slide, the presenter blanked the screen (by pressing B and return on the keyboard). When a screen goes black, the audience naturally gives all of their focus back to the presenter.

She put the slide advancer down. She looked serious as she walked toward the audience until she was close enough to touch them. She waited a few moments and began in hushed, almost whispered tones. "On October 23, 2010, at some time after midnight a warehouse at the end of the block caught fire. (pause) They think maybe homeless people attempting to withstand the desperately cold night lit a fire that got out of control. When the warehouse burned, it caused the office building next to it to burn (in the air next to her she is gesturing the position of each subsequent building) and the next and the next. (extended pause) Our clinic did not escape. Six years of dreams and (she looks down searching for the right word) sweat and *love* wiped out in a single blaze. The city's skyline glowed. The local news sent satellite trucks to cover the story.

I watched in disbelief from the tiny TV in our kitchen. Gone. Everything is gone."

I was in the audience, and I looked at the people in the room. They were all fixated, leaning forward and hanging on each word. It was a powerful moment of real connection between the presenter and the audience, and I do not think that would have happened if she had just shown another slide.

Do you need a slide? Most of the time, no. When we speak something magical happens. Our brain waves sync up. Researchers have hooked up presenters and members of the audience to MRIs and as the presenter speaks the audience begins to shadow the brain patterns. When you describe something like the fire in the previous example, you build that image *inside the person listening*, and that is powerful. That is a connection and a significant experience. The same experience told through a slide deck lacks that connection. The audience isn't working hard to imagine what the presenter is saying because they do not need to. It's shown perfectly well on an enormous screen there next to the presenter. The less *imagining work* a person does, the *less involved* they are in the process and the more distant they can be.

That said, let's talk about a few ways to make your PowerPoint better.

A time for proof

Studies show the use of a "scientific-looking" graphic makes your premise considerably more convincing. It does not matter if your graphic provides any new information; just the fact that there is a graphic dramatically improves your believability.

Early on provide one or two supporting graphics or quotes from a study. Once your audience is convinced of the veracity of your claims they'll be more likely to settle in and hear you out.

Data is beautiful

The communication benefits of sharing data are almost unmatched. We can dismiss your opinion, but we cannot deny your data. Data tells a story with the dominant force of reason. Area nine outperformed Area eight. How do we know? Look at the data. Product A is a dud while Product B flies off the shelf. Really? Yes, look at the data.

However, when data is shared on a slide quite often rather than explaining the story it obscures it. However, this is not true of printed graphs. That's because there are two tremendous disadvantages the data *slide* has compared to the data *handout*:

- Time. When we have the charts in front of us, we can peruse them as long as is necessary.
- Focus. In our hands, we can 'zoom in' to look at the data closer.

Data, complicated enough on a printed graph, becomes confounding on a slide. This, then, necessitates the absolute crystal-clear clarity of data slides.

Help your audience understand the story behind the data

What is the story your data is trying to tell? We do not collect data to have data. We collect data to understand what's going on. In that data is a story: collections are up, the census is down, and the East Side is outpacing Downtown. Elective surgeries are lagging while emergency room visits are up. Think about that story and why you would want to share it with others. Your audience begins with the question, "So what" and then ends with the question, "Now what?" What actions will we take based on the data?

An example may help to explain. A client showed us a graphic, which seemed to demonstrate the clinic was doing well and had been doing well for years. Also, yet she was concerned. "Don't you see the problem?" I must confess I did not. She pointed out the clinic's continuing growth while the town's population was shrinking. Her clinic was already a big fish in a small town. Projected growth charts had her clinic leveling off and then contracting. To maintain their current level of operation in future years, their only option was to expand to other communities. However, they had no experience launching into unknown territory, and their success would be uncertain at best. The dilemma, as she explained it, was this: do they continue to be the dominant force in that one town and be ready to constrict with the town's population, or do they expand into new areas, risking their capital investment and reputation in situations where they have no expertise. Once we understood the story, the data was trying to show; it was relatively easy to create a line graph that showed the clinic growth and the population decrease. She was able to map out a theoretical future moment when the population would no longer support a clinic of that size.

Tell the truth

Appearing to fudge the data to support your premise can be catastrophic, not just to your speech but your career.

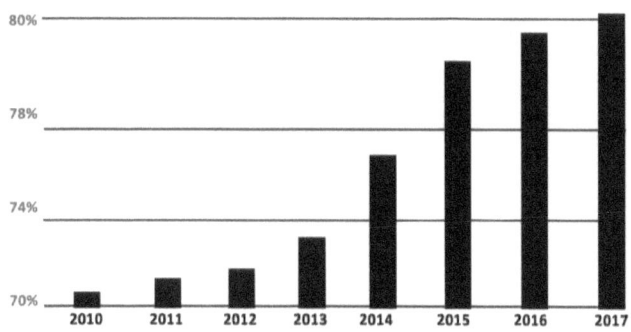

The graphic above does indeed show an increase from 70% to 80% in seven years, and that may be significant. It appears, however, to show a much more dramatic improvement. One might read it to mean in the seven years this number has gone up by a factor of ten! The graphic by itself is valid, but the accompanying explanation would almost certainly need to acknowledge the change was from seventy to eighty percent, that is, only ten percent rather than that factor of ten.

Help us to understand where to look.

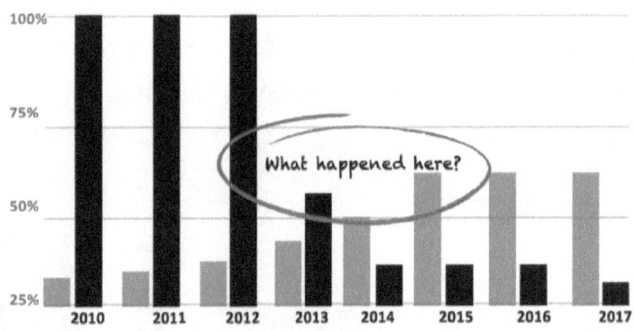

Your audience may only get a couple of minutes to examine a chart, so you may be doing them a favor to point out the essential parts of the graphic visually.

PowerPoint is not a teleprompter

I get it. You have not spent enough time to memorize your presentation permanently, so you put as much as you can on the slide deck, so you'll remember it. This *PowerPoint-as-teleprompter* cheat sheet has killed many a presentation. When every word you're saying is also on the screen, your audience is reading instead of listening. Here's a hint. If you're putting every word on slides, send your slide deck to the presentation and stay home. Most of us have been reading since we were five or six and having someone read to us is at best unnecessary and at worst condescending. Your audience can read it at their leisure instead of having you read it to them.

PowerPoint is a visual medium and works best with big images and very little text. Paragraphs of tightly-spaced words belong on a handout not on the screen. If you see a section of text anywhere in the deck, go back and condense that into one word or short phrase.

This slide merely is paragraphs of text lifted from a website. The audience would be unlikely to be able to read it.

HOMELESS VETERANS

Homeless veterans are younger on average than the total veteran population. Approximately 9% are between the ages of 18 and 30, and 41% are between the ages of 31 and 50. Conversely, only 5% of all veterans are between the ages of 18 and 30, and less than 23% are between 31 and 50.

Roughly 45% of all homeless veterans are African American or Hispanic, despite only accounting for 10.4% and 3.4% of the U.S. veteran population, respectively.

Although flawless counts are impossible to come by – the transient nature of homeless populations presents a major difficulty – the U.S. Department of Housing and Urban Development (HUD) estimates that 39,471 veterans are homeless on any given night.

A better version might look like this:

Reducing the text to a few key phrases helps, but this is still too much like a handout and does not fully utilize the power of the PowerPoint slide format.

HOMELESS VETERANS

They are younger than average veterans with 41% between ages of 31 and 50

Almost half are African American or Hispanic

Almost 40,000 veterans are homeless on any given night

This, however, is more compelling:

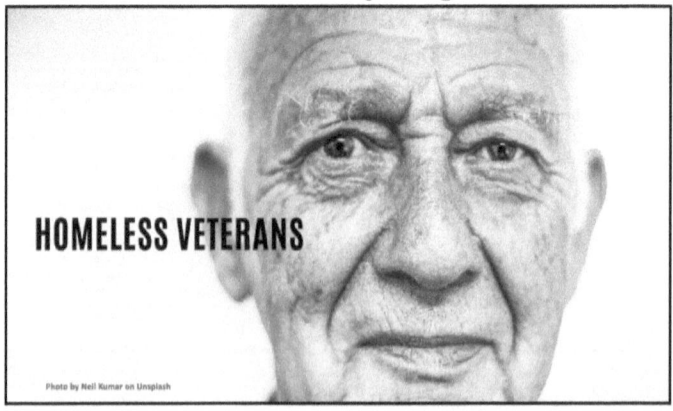

One simple large image extending beyond the borders of the screen forces us to look into the eyes of this person rather than cold statistics in a bullet point. Once this image is displayed the presenter can verbally share the same statistics. Most are between thirty-one and fifty, roughly half are African American or Hispanic, and every night about 40,000 veterans sleep on the streets. This technique is dramatically more powerful than a block of text on a white page.

Keep it simple

Choices, choices. You can fade, cut, dissolve, checkerboard, flip, flash, fly through, orbit, glitter, shred, switch, split, or zoom from one slide to another. All of these are transitions built into the PowerPoint slide software. Which ones should you use to go from one slide to another? None. Skip all the flashy transitions, animations, and sound effects. The most potent choices for almost every purpose are:

- Fade
- Cut

That's it. If you watch an evening's worth of TV or see a major motion picture, the chances are excellent that these two boring old transitions are all you'll ever see. Why? Wouldn't it be more exciting to *jelly-roll* or *confetti-bomb* from one captivating slide to another? [1]All of that flash draws attention to the wrong thing. It's like showing up at your wedding with a tie that's lit up and flashing. It would indeed be more exciting, but what a shame it would be to take the attention away from the majesty of the occasion for something so tacky and trivial.

A fade suggests the two slides are related. For instance, you might show patient satisfaction results from before, fade, and after to illustrate how things have changed. If you keep all of the information the same on both slides except the bar representing the score, a fade transition helps the audience compare and contrast. However, please, make it a short transition.

A cut is the most useful transition we can use. It suggests merely going from one idea to the next. I worked in TV for thirty-five years, and I've probably made tens of thousands of edits, and likely 99.9% of them were straight cuts. The straight cut works, the audience understands it, and it does not draw any unnecessary attention to itself.

---

[1] Jelly-roll and confetti bombs are not actual PowerPoint transitions.

I often train clients at the Studer Community Institute in Pensacola where we work with business leaders to improve their skills. Only one time have I gotten a negative comment on my training when I strongly suggested not using fancy glitter transitions between slides. This particular attendee wanted *flashing comet poofs*, and, by golly, she was going to use them. She was not at all happy I did not teach her how to create *flashing comet poofs*.[2]

Have you ever tried to talk to your kids when the TV is on? Have you noticed they could not listen to you and watch at the same time? Most people can't. So, every time you advance your slides, for a moment the audience leaves your message and turns to the PowerPoint. If the transition sparkles or swoops between slides, you'll lose your audience's attention. Restrain yourself from creating a slide deck so compelling that they look at your slides instead of at you.

Three font sizes maximum

You should use three fonts maximum. Most of the time you have a bold headline font, a medium bullet point font, and a smaller supporting font:

---

[2] Flashing comet poofs is not an actual PowerPoint transition.

HEADLINE FONT
BULLET POINT FONT
Supporting text font

The smallest font you should use is one that can be seen clearly from a point farthest from the stage in the room you will speak. A good rule of thumb is a minimum of thirty-four-point type. If possible, schedule a time to stop by the presentation room the day before and go through your presentation slides while sitting in the back row. At a minimum, bring up your PowerPoint on your computer and step away twenty feet. Can you read it clearly? If not, reduce the number of words on the screen and make the font larger.

Remember slides are designed to be read in a few seconds like you would read a billboard on the interstate. Paragraphs are unacceptable. Single words or phrases, better. One compelling image that covers the screen is best. Note the two examples below.

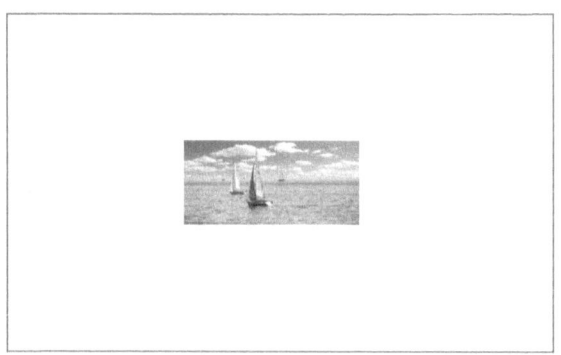

This image is too small and gets lost on the slide:

This is the same image but taken full size:

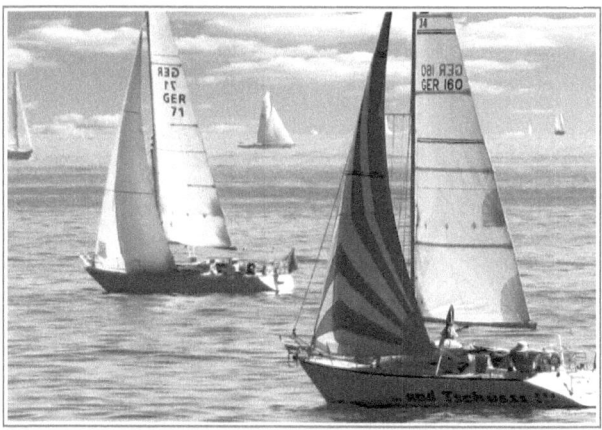

It's much more compelling when seen full screen.

If using multiple images on a screen, make sure they line up and are the same size:

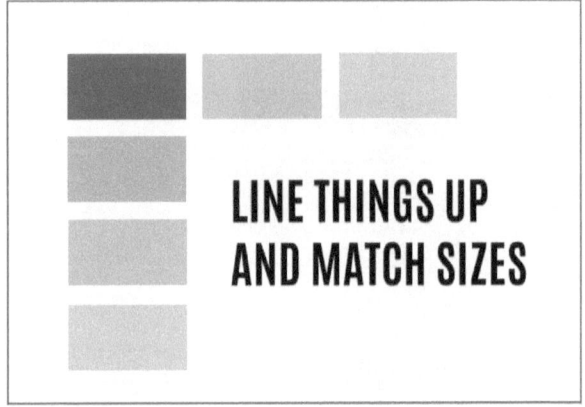

Resist the temptation to create a photo collage. Too often they just become a muddy mess. Even professional artists struggle to make a collage

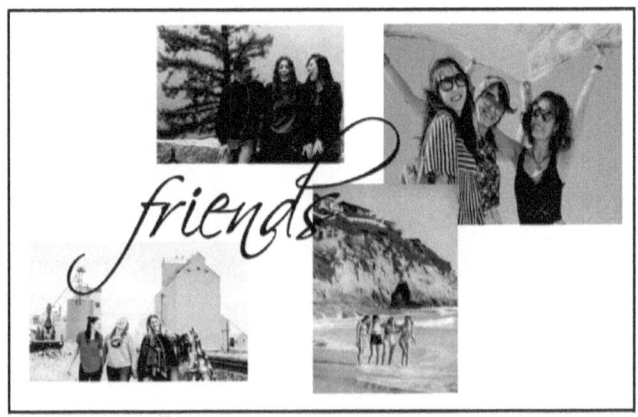

that works. One full-screen image usually has more impact than a bunch of random images thrown together. Plus, enlarge your image in what's called "full bleed," that is, run it off the screen on all sides.

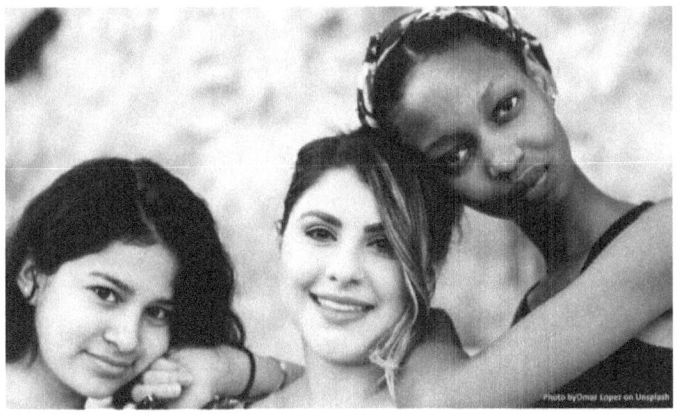

Where do you get the images? Randomly grabbing images off the Internet is not only a bad idea, but it is also illegal.

Copyright laws prohibit using another person's photos without their consent. I remember my boss's wife getting quite upset with me when I pointed that out. "But they're on the Internet already! That means you're free to use them!" Actually, no you are not. She was determined enough that she called the firm's attorney to find out and sheepishly came back and apologized.

That also goes for using hit songs. Yes, it probably would be great to start your yearly conference with "Let's Get it Started" by the Black-Eyed Peas, but without permission, you run the risk of a costly lawsuit. Also, yes, I understand you bought it on iTunes, but still, rights to own it and listen to yourself and rights to play it in a public space are different. This also goes for playing video. Grabbing a scene from *Caddy shack* might make your point but might even get you smacked with a sizeable fine.

Copyright laws are a complicated subject, and I'm not giving legal advice, I'm just trying to caution you. A phone call to your legal counsel can provide you the best answer and also give you the best protection.

So where do you get images? Stock photography has gotten much better in the past few years. At one-time stock photos looked stilted and plastic with perfect plastic people in full white offices. Now you are much more likely to find an image that looks and feels like real life. However, the best bet might be to buy a decent camera and take photos yourself, being careful, of course, to not violate HIPAA or patient privacy laws.

Also, realize the best photos may have nothing to do with healthcare. If you want to focus on customer service, you may want to take a picture of your favorite barista. To illustrate teamwork, you might consider a photo of your son's little league team. Alignment might be a photo of your daughter in the Nutcracker. Many newer smartphones can take pictures sufficient to play in a PowerPoint. Just get in the habit of taking photos everywhere.

Create your PowerPoint to optimize how it will be played.

Before you begin any presentation, make sure your PowerPoint slides are correctly set up for the monitor that will be used. There are a few technical considerations you should be aware of before you begin.

It is unfortunate that an older version of PowerPoint defaults to a four by three format.

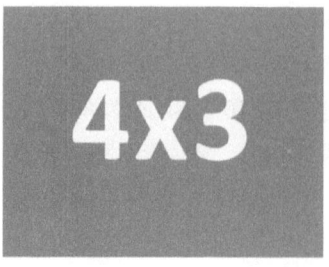

What does that mean? The screen is just a little wider than it is tall. Like this:

The fine folks at Microsoft are more interested in how the slides look on your computer than how they look on the monitor when you play them in front of a crowd. Most new monitors have screen dimensions of 16 x 9 like this:

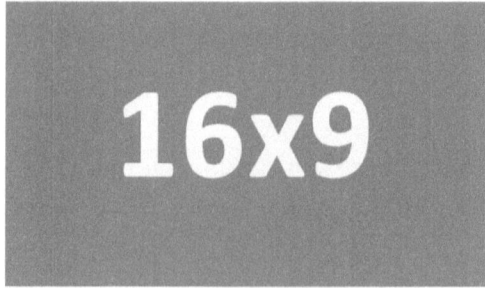

In June 2009 all American broadcasts switched from standard definition signals to high definition signals, providing dramatically better pictures, sound, and motion. They also began broadcasting in the 16x9 format.

Since then older standard definition TVs and monitors have been replaced almost everywhere with new HD TVs. Chances are good when you play your PowerPoint on a screen in the conference room; it will be played on an HD TV. What happens, though, when your 4x3 images show up on a 16x9 monitor?

This is what happens. You probably remember this from your old TV days, after the switch but before you bought your new HD TV.

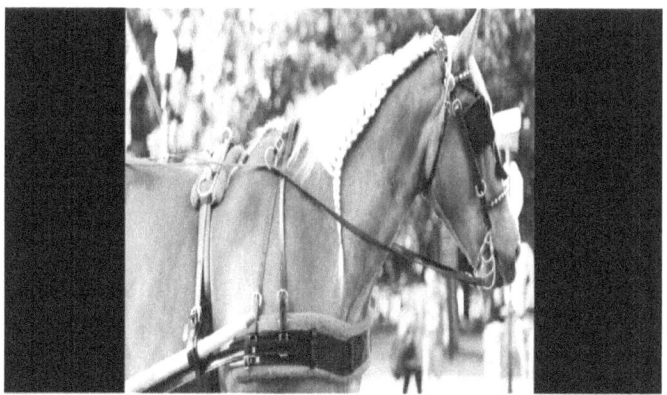

The image will be stretched, and these ugly bars will appear down either side.

To avoid that, before you begin creating your first slide do this:

1. Go to file, page setup

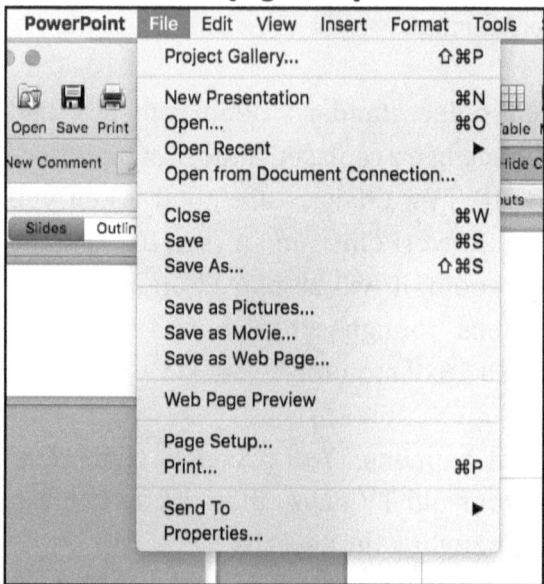

2. Select on-screen show (16:9)

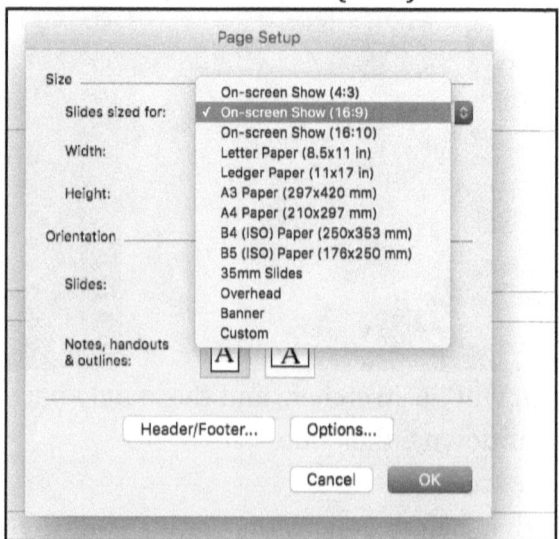

Now when you build your slideshow, it will be optimized for the monitors you play it on. If you have questions about the format of the room in which you'll be presenting, check with your AV team. They'll understand all of this and will help guide you to the best format.

Your AV team will also know whether your PowerPoint program is the latest version. Sometimes slides created on an older version look distorted when they are played on the newest version. Getting your slides back on track can take some time, and that's not a worry you need moments before your presentation.

Given a choice, you should always choose to play your presentation on the same computer that created it. That often means nothing more than plugging your laptop into the monitor or projector. Before building a complete slide deck, though, ask if you are following someone else or if you cannot plug your computer into the system. Primarily if you cannot use your computer, you want to make sure, ahead of time, which your slides work well and look good on the other system. Several days beforehand, try out your slides on the very equipment you will use. If you have to make adjustments, you want plenty of time to do so, something you cannot do in the hour or two before your presentation. Try not to "Just send them, and we'll get our guys to look." Other people may not realize when some part of a slide is cut off, or if a font is different.

Many times, your organization has an approved template. In that case, of course, you'll want to create a compliant slide deck. Still, format it for 16x9 before you begin so it will look best on the monitor.

Too important to be left to an intern

Leaders often work for weeks on preparing a perfect presentation, only to hand off their PowerPoint to an intern to prepare. That's a shame. Your impact will be dramatically better if you take the design of your graphics seriously. If we have a monetary investment and reputation on the line, we can destroy it with poorly crafted slides.

Ask your art department to get involved. If you do not have access to an art department and this is a big presentation, it may be time to hire an agency or graphic design firm to help. However, make sure the team you hire knows presentation software. Ask to see samples and get referrals before you hire them. The skills required to do good print work are not the same as the skills needed to create beautiful slides. Showing up with bad graphics is equivalent to showing up in an ill-fitting, wrinkled suit. What a shame if you let a single presentation with poorly prepared visuals damage your reputation with the organization.

PowerPoint, Keynote, and Prezi

You may wonder why I have not mentioned other slide presentation programs like Keynote and Prezi. I am a Mac fan, I am writing this on a Mac, my wife has a Mac, and we've had a series of iPhones through the years. The biggest challenge with Keynote is that not everyone uses it. Many times, I cannot determine ahead of time which computer will be used to present the slideshow. I'm grateful when it is mine because I have both Keynote and PowerPoint. However, often you won't know which computer will be used until the last moment. You can export a Keynote slide deck into a PowerPoint format, but it almost always distorts the slides. Things run off the screen here and there, and fonts show up distorted. Transitions do not work at all. This is not a headache you need minutes before a presentation. PowerPoint is the default slide presentation software, and you are always safest to start there.

Prezi is cool, but that is also its downside. You zoom in on a topic, word or image and then on the next click, you zoom back. Cool, right? Unfortunately, people are so taken by the software that they no longer are paying attention to the speaker.

One final thought. If you give many presentations, it might make sense to buy your slide advancer. I like the Kensington Wireless Presenter. It's simple, with forward and back buttons and 'blank the screen' button. Blanking the screen is used for the time you do not want the slide to be up there. On a computer keyboard you can hit 'B' and return, and it does the same thing.

Making sense of diagrams

Diagrams and charts do wonders to make complex information understandable:

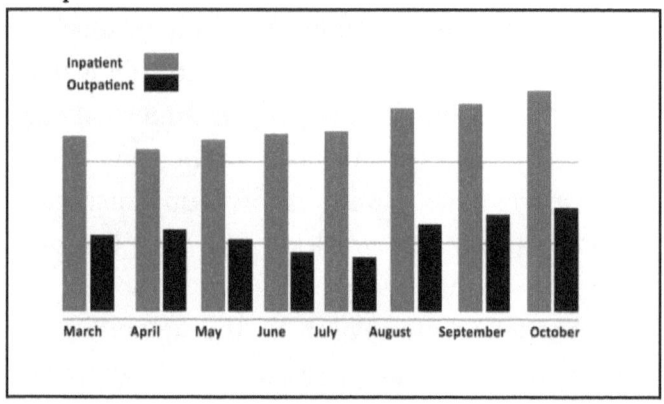

A well-made chart will give your audience a split-second snapshot of the data. There are, however, a few precautions to consider.

Use the right chart for the correct data

Pie charts are useful for showing how each percentage compares to the whole. If you're comparing the company's profits across regions, it's a quick snapshot to see how each division compares to others. Pie charts can be limiting as they work for only a few data sets with reasonably large differences between that data.

Pie charts illustrate a few sets quite well

If instead, we were comparing twenty-four data sets, the slices would be too small to be meaningful:

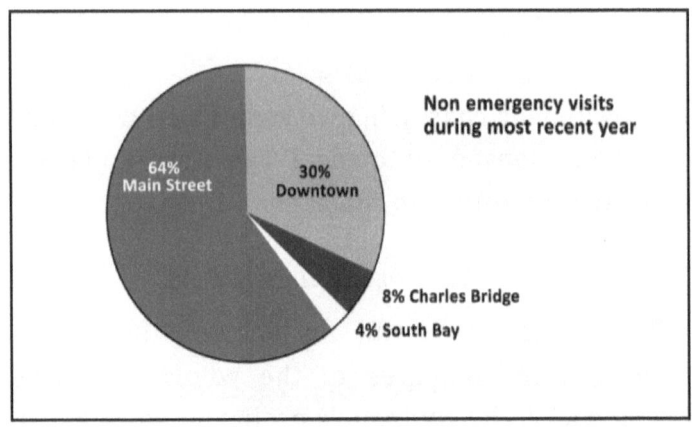

Bar charts are better for showing large data sets that have smaller differences

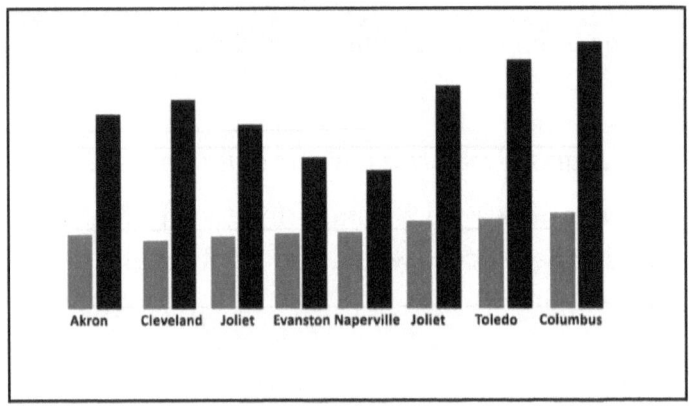

Line graphs help us understand change over time.

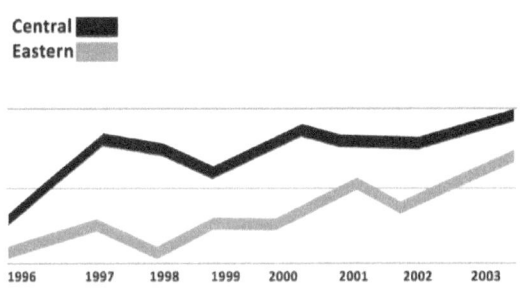

communicating it.

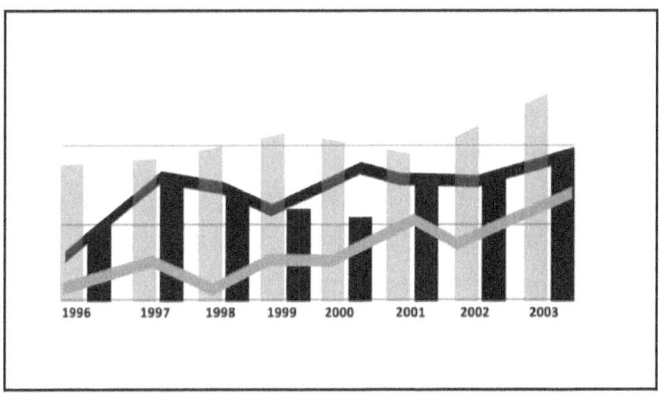

Your goal is to clarify your data, not to obscure it. When you pop up a slide and say, "I know you can't read this very well," you have failed. If the data is too dense, create more than one slide. Remove all information that isn't essential for your audience to understand. Work with high contrast colors and simple fonts. Make sure your fonts can be read from across the room. The only reason to include a chart is to make the data more accessible to understand. Ask someone to review your slides. If they are not legible or do not make sense, re-work the images until they are solid.

Your slide deck provides a sequence, so each slide builds on the one before it. Remember, no one slide has to do it all. Think of slides as a sequence of thoughts, one following another:

- Slide one shows expected census of four quarters
- Switch to slide two to show the actual census over the four quarters
- You ask, "Well? What happened?"
- Switch to slide three that shows your key market areas and one area that is down considerably
- Slide four divides your crucial market areas into individual centers to explain how the downtown census plummeted in the final two quarters

This is a powerful way to use your data to convey a complicated story over a series of slides rather than trying to communicate everything on one slide that gets too busy.

Bonus Chapter

Dress for Success

The purpose of your presentation is to help your audience, sometimes through inspiration, other times through education, but always with the focus on elevating the audience. The gift you're bringing is a well-crafted presentation, and the journey you're taking them on is meant to be enjoyed. Throughout this book, we've sought to remove barriers to engagement and to enhance your audience's ability to listen, understand, and accept your message. A poor outfit choice on your part can wreck all of that hard work.

Dressing for success during a presentation means studiously removing anything from your outfit that distracts from your message. If they're noticing only your outfit, they're not noticing your message. I found that out all too well in Atlanta. I felt like I'd given an engaging workshop and, when we were through, a dozen attendees lined up to chat with me. Unfortunately, the message I heard three different times was, "I love your tie!" They noticed the bright orange tie I was wearing and that was enough to distract them from my presentation. That is what failure to dress for success looks like.

> *If they notice what you are wearing instead of seeing your message you have failed to dress for success.*

Tina, a bright young presenter, gave a beautifully-crafted breakout session at a major conference, but her last-minute decision to wear bright red pumps meant the audience noticed her outfit and forgot her main points. Carolyn, a skilled nurse leader, would have wowed the audience at her annual conference, but her loose, floppy, wildly colorful outfit eroded her credibility and sank her effectiveness.

Dressing for success on the stage means almost always dressing more conservatively than you do anywhere else. In fact, if we went to most conferences and tried to guess ahead of time that the main speakers were, we could pick them out because they would be dressed better and more conservatively than the rest of the crowd. At many conferences, the only people wearing suits are the keynote speakers.

So why all the charcoal suits? Conservative clothing looks neat and attractive but does not call attention to oneself. We tend to think the woman in the dark suit and the white blouse looks smart or intelligent. Her outfit enhances her credibility. Quint Studer told me, "A suit means you take this presentation seriously." While overall, we've seen office norms slide toward the more and more casual side, top presenters still wear traditional gray, navy, or black suits with white or blue shirts or stylish but straightforward, dark-colored dresses. Because women have so many more options in their clothing choices, selecting the conservative dress or suit is usually the best approach. At some conferences, the tie has become optional for men, but it's always safest to wear one and take it off later.

You might assume a formally-outfitted presenter seems less approachable to a casually-dressed audience, and that is indeed true, but the conservative outfit gives us much-needed credibility right from the start. How much more difficult for the presenter in jeans and a t-shirt which has to spend much of his talk building credibility. The woman in the perfect suit can build her connection with the audience throughout her speech, telling self-deprecating stories and confessing I'm-just-like-you weaknesses. She has the opportunity to do this because she is not working to establish her credibility.

Conservative, by the way, does not mean any dark suit or dress will do. The fit is more important than cost. A moderately-priced outfit with perfect fit trumps a lavish outfit that is too big or too small for you. A few dollars at a tailor can be money well spent.

Conservative means avoiding the trends. When you scan the local fashion magazines, and they scream, "Chartreuse, your color to <u>wow</u> this year," run away as quickly as you can. Skinny jeans are for baristas, not business leaders. Facebook founder Mark Zuckerberg became a millionaire and then started wearing t-shirts on stage at major events, not the other way around.

Conservative does not mean wearing a suit you bought when Ronald Reagan was President. We've seen way too many men in their fifties and sixties wearing out of date suits and ties. "It still fits, and I'm going to wear it," can be damaging to your credibility. As we get later in our careers especially in industries that lean toward younger people, more mature people have to work extra hard to maintain their relevance. First impressions matter. Go to a top-end men's clothing store and look at their suits. There are subtle but significant differences that make a new suit appear fresh and up to date.

Anything revealing is distracting. A hint of cleavage is enough to sidetrack your message, as is a tight skirt or spike heels. Your goal in this presentation is to make a difference and not to get a date. If there is a doubt, leave it out. A good guideline would be to watch the main anchors on the news, Robin Roberts, Ann Curry, Katie Couric, and Diane Sawyer. Look at what they wear while delivering the news and copy it. Wear less jewelry than you think, and make sure it's not dangly, bright, or distracting. Men should probably not wear any jewelry beyond a classic watch and a wedding ring. Jewelry can catch stage lights and glint as you move around, distracting from your message.

No matter what you wear make sure it is cleaned and pressed. If you are traveling to this event, you may need to call your hotel ahead of time to make sure you have a steam iron in your room. Take a spare of everything just in case you spill coffee or break a heel off at the last minute.

Men, please get rid of all the stuff from your pockets. Cell phones can play havoc with your wireless microphones. Make sure they are turned off, not just silent, and stowed away in a briefcase back at your seat or with a friend. Wallets, keys, breath mints, pens, change can all destroy your silhouette, making a great suit look lumpy.

Your personal brand

Chances are you already have a personal brand. A personal brand is the total of ways other people see you. It's your style, your manner, and your approach to things. Oprah has a brand, Sir Richard Branson has a brand, and Matthew McConaughey has a brand. All three people have a particular 'look' and a way of approaching the world that sets them apart.

In any discussion about dressing for success, we would be remiss if we did not discuss your own personal brand. Are you casual or formal? Are you approachable or reserved? Are you witty or intellectual? Answering these questions can inform how you dress for success.

Recently, when I was hired to train at a children's hospital, the chief of endocrinology shared an elevator with me. "We do not wear suits around here," he said, eyeing my navy two-button, "and we certainly *do not* wear ties." With that, he flipped my tie up and away and stepped off the elevator. I knew what he meant, but I also knew the power of a personal brand. This is what *my brand* looks like and maintaining my particular brand is more important than complying with some unspoken dress code.

If you try too hard to fit in, you may well be forgotten. My friend Ann almost always wears robin's-egg blue to match her eyes. It is her personal branded color, and anyone can pick her out of a crowd. President Barack Obama wore a simple dark suit and a white shirt every day for the eight years he was President. It was such a personal brand that one day when he wore a tan suit, the news media lit up with stories about it.

Personal branding goes beyond what you wear, but what you wear has to fit your approach to life. Simon Sinek is smart, approachable and casual. His clothing choices match that. Jackie Kennedy, and indeed all of the Kennedys, were well known for an unexpected elegance in American political circles.

Pick a style that suits you and then do not deviate. Branding is really about being consistent. Coke, one of the most valuable brands in history, is always associated with red, indeed, Pantone 484. The company spends millions every year making sure the red you see on their products in Peru or Pakistan exactly matches the red you see on their bottles in Pulaski.

All of This is Worthless

We have covered a lot in this book, but we want you to understand that all of this is worthless. You have wasted your time. You should have done something else. This is of no value to you or anyone else... that is... unless you put it into practice. If you attend our class, read the book and set it aside, you will not have benefited at all.

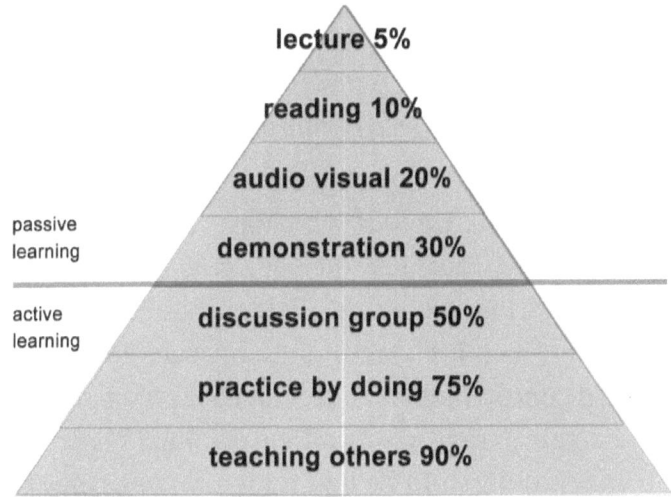

Source: National Training Laboratories, Bethel Maine

We all know you cannot learn to roller-skate by reading a book or ride a bicycle by watching someone else do so on TV. Speaking is a physical act. You have to *do it to* get better. So here is a secret: we are all terrible at first. The expert, the one you admire so much, was awful, absolutely atrocious at the beginning. You have to be willing to be bad first, to try and fail, over and over again.

Remember the good news

Most people grow to be incredibly better speakers in a short period. If you find yourself held back and not progressing as rapidly as others, you likely fall into one of these categories:

You did not memorize your presentation

During one of my classes, a bright young man puzzled me. He was articulate, his content was organized, but his delivery was wooden and uninspiring. It became evident that he had never memorized his nine-minute speech. Four weeks had gone by, and he could not speak from memory a single paragraph. I politely declined to continue his training until he had it memorized. Once that happened he immediately became a very different presenter. He was able to work on gestures, tone and pausing because he was no longer struggling with pure memorization.

You've always been a "High-B Student."
Most of us know two or three people who are just great at everything they do. They can take a test without studying and still make a solid grade. They're funny, likable, the real life of the party. These people, the ones I call the High-B Student, are frustrating to work with because they do well by exerting minimal effort.

They never buckle down and do the hard work. If they are already getting a "High-B" without practice, what incentive do they have to spend hours working on their presentation? A "High-B Student" can become exceptional, but only if they put forth maximum effort and do the hard work that it takes to excel.

You are not paying attention to your audience
I've worked with the occasional business leaders who like to hear themselves talk. Their audience is not consequential to them and could go to sleep, pass out or leave. They would never think to vary their presentation. Don't be like them, forgetting that your audience is the reason for your presentation. If you cannot engage your audience and keep them engaged, it is your fault. Start by studying as much as you can about your audience before you present. If possible send out a pre-conference survey. At the very least, poll the

audience about their concerns before you begin your presentation.

Final Thoughts

The Space Shuttle, I've been told, was *off target eighty-four percent* of the time. That is, its trajectory was incorrect, and its direction flawed. If it continued on that path, it would not reach its objective. Luckily it had onboard a device that sent a little "ping" to Earth every few minutes. The space center back on Earth would send a "ping" back to the shuttle so it could alter its path and for another few minutes be on target.

That's what we need to do with our audience. Send out a ping. Say, "Have you ever been lost?" *Ping.* Then observe our audiences. Alternatively, say, "Does this make sense?" We look to see if our audience responds. *Ping.* If we do this, we can alter our paths and for the next few minutes be back on target.

I'd love to hear from you, so I'm sending out my own "ping." My email address is:

DanielPennington@Speaker-Training.org

Tell me what you enjoyed learning and what you would like to learn more about next time.

I wish you every success!

Speaking Checklist

Here are a few questions to ask yourself or to ask the person watching you practice. Answer them truthfully:

1. Did you make eye contact before you began? How was your eye contact throughout?

2. Did you capture the audience's attention from the first line?

3. How was the pace of the speech? Too slow? Too fast?

4. Did you vary your tone/volume/pace several times in the speech?

5. Did you use pauses? Did you extend pauses to three or four seconds or more?

6. How much did your audience learn from this speech? What were the key takeaways?

7. Could the audience repeat the central theme after listening and watching?

8. Were there enough examples to make sure everything was clear?

9. Were there any words that the average person on the street would struggle to understand?

10. Was there any jargon in the speech? Unexplained acronyms?

11. Was each step in the journey satisfying?

12. Were there any questions left unanswered?

13. Did it sound conversational?

14. Were you able to paint vibrant word pictures for your audience?

15. What mental images will your audience have stuck in their heads?

16. Were the attempts at humor natural or a little awkward? Was there enough humor?

17. Did you notice any annoying traits? Throat clearing?

18. Did your hand gestures and body posture enforce your words or detract from your point?

19. If someone watched the speech with the sound
off would they still have some idea of the tone?

20. Were there annoying words or phrases like,
   "you know," or "well, basically?"

21. Did the presentation feel too long or too short?

22. Was the audience ever a little confused?

23. Was the audience ever a bit bored?

24. Did you ever feel emotionally moved by the content? Did your audience?

25. Was the information fresh or have others already covered this topic?

26. Did you finish strong?

27. Did you use active language?

28. Were you clear on what you want the audience to think, do, or feel as a result of this presentation?

29. Did you mention how your audience might obtain more information?

Acknowledgments

I am lucky to be surrounded by some of the smartest people I know. My wife, Donna, and daughter, Isadora, have been crucial to the success of this project. Many of the initial ideas and processes contained in this book have initially been fleshed out by them. Early versions were edited and proofed by Isadora and Donna before this became a real book.

The ever-patient Marilyn Oberhausen has provided editorial assistance. Without her eagle eyes and exhaustive attention to detail, this book would not be where it is today.

My colleague and friend Rachael Gillette has been a steadfast promoter of this work from the beginning. She was instrumental in employing me as faculty with the Studer Community Institute, which began my independent training career. Her counsel in this process has been invaluable.

My association with Quint Studer has dramatically improved my life and those of many others. He is a friend and mentor, and there is no way I could have accomplished much of this without his help and guidance.

Also, I am most thankful for my clients. They've trusted us to push them out of their comfort zones and make them do things they never thought they could do. Every day I am amazed at how hard they work, how focused they have become, and how ready they are to stretch themselves and their abilities. I may be the coach, but they are my heroes. Thank you for trusting our process and sharing a part of your dream with us.

About the Author

Daniel began his career in Nashville at the largest film company in Tennessee. As the producer, he worked on national commercials with clients like GMC, KFC, Kraft Foods, Shoney's, and John Deere.

From there he was recruited to WVEC-TV in Virginia Beach, where, as Art Director, he developed graphics packages for many regional Belo TV stations.

Along the way, he found time to write and illustrate two children's books.

Returning to Nashville, Daniel was hired to create a new look and promotional branding for WSMV-TV, the flagship station in the Meredith Corporation. Alongside a team of top executives Daniel ensured, WSMV was the number one most watched TV station for eight years. For their efforts, the team was finalists for the Regional Emmy awards.

Always a beach lover, in 2002 Daniel jumped at the chance to work at WEAR-TV and gratefully found himself living on the sugar white sand beaches of Pensacola, Florida. Daniel directed a

team of video professionals to create cutting-edge television
programs, commercials, and news products to enhance the Sinclair brand. His team racked up an impressive list of Addy Awards along the way; helping more than ten thousand businesses learn to present their products and services through the medium of television.

In 2010 Daniel joined the Studer Group as a Communication Specialist where he worked extensively with Studer Group's top speakers and presenters. Along the way, he began training new speakers and subject matter experts on how to present their content effectively.

Now as an independent consultant, Daniel works with local and national firms to enhance their executives' presentation skills. In one-on-one training and small group exercises, Daniel can help almost any presenter improve these valuable skills.

Daniel Pennington's Speaker Training

Over the years we've developed a system that works. While every speaker is different, and every situation is different, most training classes end up looking like one of these options. Inevitably we build the training around you, your team, your challenges, and your goals.

Speaker Training Workshops. A workshop can last from two hours to an entire eight-hour day but generally begins with a lecture followed by hands-on training. For those who do not have much time, these can communicate critical information and offer real-life practice at the same time. The limitation is that workshops lack the repetition of learning available in other choices. Best for group sizes from a handful to a roomful.

Speaker Training Small Groups. Bring your team together to learn in our small group settings. Organizations that train together attain critical alignment and learn to coordinate their messages and maximize their impact. This four-step training plan focuses the first two training session on constructing a message with impact and the second two training sessions on how to deliver that message. Each session utilizes videotaped feedback to allow participants to validate their progress. These sessions work best for small groups of four to ten employees.

Speaker Training One-on-One. One-on-one training is the single most effective process for achieving results. Daniel works with the leader to carefully construct a message, delivery, body language, vocal tone and stage presence. This four-stage training process is completed through a series of training sessions that are videotaped and analyzed minute-by-minute to make you the best presenter you can be.

© 2018 Daniel Pennington

All rights reserved. This book or parts thereof may not be reproduced in any form, stored in any retrieval system, or transmitted in any form by any means—electronic, mechanical, photocopy, recording, or otherwise—without prior written permission of the publisher, except as provided by United States of America copyright law.

For permission requests, write to the publisher, at "Attention: Permissions Coordinator," at the address below.
www.speaker-training.org
1289 East Avery, Pensacola FL 32503

To order more books or coaching requests
Call (850) 400-6115

www.ingramcontent.com/pod-product-compliance
Lightning Source LLC
Chambersburg PA
CBHW031614210526
45464CB00004B/1574

HOW TO GET ON MORE PODCASTS...

AND GROW YOUR BUSINESS

By Lindsay Reid